FOR

FORK'S

SAKE

RACHAEL J BROWN

FOR
FORK'S
SAKE

A QUICK GUIDE TO HEALING YOURSELF AND
THE PLANET THROUGH A PLANT-BASED DIET

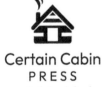

Certain Cabin
PRESS
www.forforkssakebook.com

ISBN: 979-8-9861380-0-8 (ebook)
ISBN: 979-8-9861380-1-5 (paperback)
ISBN: 979-8-9861380-2-2 (hardcover)

Ordering Information:
Special discounts are available on quantity purchases by corporations, associations, and others. For details, contact forforkssakebook@gmail.com or visit www.forforkssakebook.com.

To anyone who has wanted to make changes but felt overwhelmed by all the health information out there, I hope this helps.

And,

To my husband and kids who tried the chard smoothie and lived to tell about it, thanks for learning with me. May you always remember:
YOU'RE GETTING ENOUGH PROTEIN.

TABLE OF CONTENTS

"Nutrition is the master key to human health."
—T. Colin Campbell, PhD[1]

DAY 0

FROM TEN YEARS TO TEN DAYS

TWELVE YEARS AGO, my then five-year-old nephew was diagnosed with cancer. At the time, his mom was in nursing school, and a professor asked her if she'd looked at the role of nutrition in cancer and suggested a few books. My sister-in-law took this advice to heart, and in a very short period of time went from eating pork and chicken that she'd raised to eating vegan and juicing.

Understand, this was the same woman who'd inspired me to buy a cheese-making kit and taught me how to pull mozzarella a year earlier. Amazed by the changes she'd made in such a short time—and because of her transformation—I began reading the suggested books too.

Next, I started watching documentaries and did other research. The more I found out, the more I realized I needed to change my eating habits. I had personal reasons for wanting to make changes. High cholesterol ran in our family. I'd tried for

1   T. Colin Campbell, *Whole: Rethinking the Science of Nutrition* (Dallas: BenBella Books, 2014), xii.

years to keep it under control with diet and exercise (with varying degrees of success), only to have it creep back up again. I didn't want to take cholesterol medication if I didn't have to; I'd watched my dad change cholesterol medication many times after losing his sense of taste or having some other odd side effect. My grandparents had strokes and heart attacks. My paternal grandfather had Alzheimer's and died of pancreatic cancer, as did my uncle. I had plenty of reasons to make myself as healthy as possible.

Our food is killing us

The top two killers in America, according to the CDC, are heart disease and cancer. Also in the top 10 are stroke, Alzheimer's, and diabetes[2]—all of which are diseases affected by the "Standard American Diet" or appropriately…SAD.[3]

A book called *The China Study* provided me the basis for new ways of looking at the role of diet in health. The author, Dr. T. Colin Campbell, found that genetics was not the main factor in whether someone got cancer. Initially, doing work in the Philippines to help feed hungry children, Dr. Campbell started to notice that children of wealthier families who were eating high amounts of animal protein had higher rates of liver cancer. Most importantly, Dr. Campbell later found that by changing the amounts of animal protein fed to rats, he could turn on and turn off cancer growth in tumors.[4]

2   "Leading Causes of Death," Centers for Disease Control, updated January 13, 2022, https://www.cdc.gov/nchs/fastats/leading-causes-of-death.htm.

3   "Standard American Diet," NutritionFacts.org, accessed February 27, 2022, https://nutritionfacts.org/topics/standard-american-diet/.

4   T. Colin Campbell, *The China Study: The Most Comprehensive Study of Nutrition Ever Conducted and the Startling Implications for Diet, Weight Loss, and Long-term Health* (Dallas: BenBella Books, 2006).

This was aha moment number one for me. I was thrilled to find out that my genetics weren't the main determinant of whether or not I would get cancer. Why did I not know this? Why didn't everybody know this?

I was in my mid-thirties and many people I knew were getting cancer. I wasn't sure if it was because I was getting older or noticing more, but it seemed like every month someone else was diagnosed with some sort of cancer. If animal protein feeds cancer cells, then what were we supposed to eat?

It was time.

Whole foods. Plant based. No oil. (WFPBNO)

I decided to adopt WFPBNO to guide my food choices. I will go into great detail in later chapters as to what WFPBNO means and how to transition your present eating style to this new way of eating, but in a nutshell, WFPBNO is exactly what it sounds like: **Whole Foods**, as in foods that are as minimally processed as possible (so, actual corn rather than corn chips, whole potatoes rather than potato chips),[5] **Plant-Based**, as in foods that are plants rather than animals,[6] and **No Oil**. You eat from a huge assortment of veggies, fruits, nuts, and beans, and you remove oils. Remove animal products like meat and dairy and you're most of the way there.[7]

---

5   Elaine Magee, "The Whole Foods Diet," WebMD, accessed February 27, 2022, https://www.webmd.com/food-recipes/features/the-whole-foods-diet.
6   Katherine D. McManus, "What Is a Plant-based Diet and Why Should You Try It?" Harvard Health Publishing, https://www.health.harvard.edu/blog/what-is-a-plant-based-diet-and-why-should-you-try-it-2018092614760.
7   "Living a Whole-Food, Plant-Based Life," T. Colin Campbell Center for Nutrition Studies, updated May 30 2019, https://nutritionstudies.org/whole-food-plant-based-diet-guide/.

This isn't a "diet" or a set of complicated meal plans you have to follow. It's much simpler than that. Together, we'll find foods and recipes that will become new favorites. Likely many of the things you enjoy now you'll still be able to enjoy with a few tweaks. Are you gluten-free? No problem. Where I suggest whole wheat pasta feel free to use lentil, chickpea or your favorite gluten-free pasta. Same goes for breads.

When I initially made the switch, the first question people asked me was if my family would be able to get enough protein from plants. This is still the number one question I get from people when they find out we eat only plants. Quick question: who do you personally know who is protein deficient? No one? Me neither. But people still ask.

The short answer is, you'll be getting plenty of healthy protein since the eight to 10 percent recommended dietary allowance of protein,[8] is easily and naturally provided by a WFPBNO diet.[9] For instance, broccoli has more protein than beef per calorie.[10] One cup of green peas provides 17 percent of your daily value of protein;[11] a cup of cooked spinach contains 11 percent of the daily value;[12] a cup of cooked large white beans provides 35 percent;[13] one cup of cooked greens—think kale,[14] Swiss

8   T. Colin Campbell, "The Mystique of Protein and Its Implications," T. Colin Campbell Center for Nutrition Studies, January 3, 2019, https://nutritionstudies. org/mystique-of-protein-implications/.

9   Ibid.

10   "Scott Stoll, "Yes, Plants Have Protein," January 15, 2013, https://www. wholefoodsmarket.com/tips-and-ideas/archive/yes-plants-have-protein.

11   "Cooked Green Peas," My Food Data, accessed February 24, 2022, https://tools. myfooddata.com/nutrition-facts/170420/wt1/1.

12   "Cooked Spinach," My Food Data, accessed February 24, 2022, https://tools. myfooddata.com/nutrition-facts/168463/wt1/1.

13   "Cooked Large White Beans," My Food Data, accessed February 24, 2022, https:// tools.myfooddata.com/nutrition-facts/175203/wt1/1.

14   "Cooked Kale," My Food Data, accessed February 25, 2022, https://tools. myfooddata.com/nutrition-facts/169238/wt1/1.

chard,[15] mustard[16] and collard greens—contains between 5 and 10 percent; and 23 almonds contain 12 percent of your daily value of protein.[17]

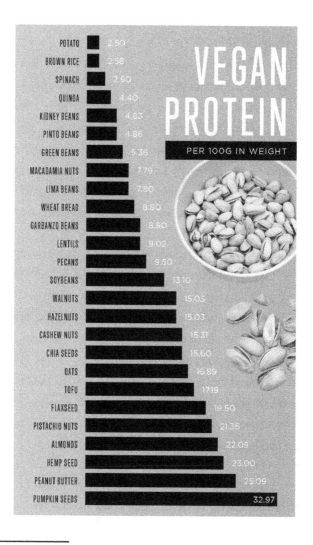

VEGAN PROTEIN

PER 100G IN WEIGHT

Food	Protein
POTATO	2.50
BROWN RICE	2.58
SPINACH	2.90
QUINOA	4.40
KIDNEY BEANS	4.83
PINTO BEANS	4.86
GREEN BEANS	5.36
MACADAMIA NUTS	7.79
LIMA BEANS	7.80
WHEAT BREAD	8.80
GARBANZO BEANS	8.90
LENTILS	9.02
PECANS	9.50
SOYBEANS	13.10
WALNUTS	15.03
HAZELNUTS	15.03
CASHEW NUTS	15.31
CHIA SEEDS	15.60
OATS	16.89
TOFU	17.19
FLAXSEED	19.50
PISTACHIO NUTS	21.35
ALMONDS	22.09
HEMP SEED	23.00
PEANUT BUTTER	25.09
PUMPKIN SEEDS	32.97

15   "Swiss Chard," My Food Data, accessed February 25, 2022, https://tools. myfooddata.com/nutrition-facts/170401/wt1/1.

16   "Mustard Greens," My Food Data, accessed February 25, 2022, https://tools. myfooddata.com/nutrition-facts/169257/wt1/1.

17   "Almonds," My Food Data, accessed February 24, 2022, https://tools.myfooddata. com/nutrition-facts/170567/wt5/1.

It's not just your family, it's everyone's family

So far I've only talked about the benefit of food to you and the health of your family. There is another beneficiary: the Earth.

In her book, *Why We Love Dogs, Eat Pigs, and Wear Cows: an Introduction to Carnism*, Melanie Joy, PhD talks about the environmental costs of carnism (a term she coined to label the belief system that conditions us to eat certain animals, like pigs, instead of, say, golden retrievers). Even back in 2006, she states, "the United Nations declared the livestock sector 'one of the top two or three most significant contributors to the most serious environmental problems, at every scale from local to global.' The UN warned, 'The impact is so significant that it needs to be addressed with urgency.'"[18]

As the world grapples with how to keep the Earth's temperature from rising, reducing our meat consumption has been found to be one of the most effective strategies. Melanie Joy continues, "In 2019, an international commission of 11,000 scientists proclaimed that people around the world must shift to a plant-focused (largely vegan) diet in order to help avert a global environmental catastrophe. Animal agriculture is one of the top three contributors to water pollution. The main sources of the pollution are antibiotics and hormones, chemicals from tanneries, animal wastes, sediments from eroded pastures, and fertilizers and pesticides used for feed crops."[19, 20]

The runoff from animal agriculture seeps into local creeks and rivers and has led to dead zones in the ocean—places where

---

18 Melanie Joy, *Why We Love Dogs, Eat Pigs, and Wear Cows: An Introduction to Carnism* (Newburyport, MA: Red Wheel, 2011), 76, 171.
19 Ibid., 77, 171.
20 William J. Ripple, Christopher Wolf, Thomas M. Newsome, et al., "World Scientists' Warning of a Climate Emergency," *BioScience* 70, no. 1 (2020): 8-12, https://doi.org/10.1093/biosci/biz088.

the oxygen levels are brought so low by pollution that plants and animals cannot survive. And it's not just the water pollution that is concerning but the amount of water used as well. As *Business Insider* put it, "A whopping 106 gallons of water goes into making just one ounce of beef."[21, 22]

The Amazon rainforest acts as a sponge and absorbs carbon dioxide that would otherwise be released into the atmosphere, contributing to global warming. However, according to Melanie Joy, "Over 75 percent of previously forested land in the Amazon has been converted into pastures for feeding farmed animals."[23]

You may have heard about antibiotics becoming resistant because of misuse or less effective because of their overuse.[24] Antibiotics are added to animal feeds in large factory farms, or CAFOs (concentrated animal feeding operations) to prevent disease in overcrowded conditions, treat infections, and improve growth and production. According to *Livestock's Long Shadow*, "in the United States…livestock are responsible for an estimated…37 percent of pesticide use [and] 50 percent of antibiotic use."[25, 26] You read that right, 50 percent of all antibiotics used in the U.S. are used in animal factory farms.

According to Melanie Joy, "Farmed animals must consume 2,000 pounds of grain in order to produce enough carnistic

21 Erin Brodwin, "One Chart Sums Up the Real Problem in the California Drought—and It Isn't Almonds," *Business Insider,* April 13, 2015, https://www.businessinsider.com/real-villain-in-the-california-drought-isnt-almonds--its-red-meat-2015-4.
22 Joy, *Why We Love Dogs, Eat Pigs, and Wear Cows,* 77, 172.
23 Joy, *Why We Love Dogs, Eat Pigs, and Wear Cows,* 77, 172.
24 "Antibiotic Resistance," World Health Organization, July 31, 2020, https://www.who.int/news-room/fact-sheets/detail/antibiotic-resistance.
25 Henning Steinfeld, Pierre Gerber, Tom Wassenaar, et al., *Livestock's Long Shadow: Environmental Issues and Options* (Rome: Food and Agriculture Organization of the United Nations, 2006), xxii.
26 Joy, *Why We Love Dogs, Eat Pigs, and Wear Cows,* 77, 172.

products to feed a person for a year. However, if that person ate the grains directly, it would take only 400 pounds of grain to feed them for a year."[27] By skipping the meat, we are also saving water and crops that go into "making" that meat. In fact, as a comparison, one five-ounce serving of beef uses 36 square miles of land and 570 gallons of water[28] and necessitates 10.50 miles driven as compared to one ¼-cup serving beans, which uses 0.15 square miles of land and 21 gallons of water with 0.11 miles driven. And how about cheese? One one-ounce serving of cheese uses 0.17 square miles of land, 37 gallons of water, and 0.60 miles driven as compared to one one-ounce serving of Kite Hill Plant-Based Cheese, which uses 0.09 square miles of land and 16 gallons of water and 0.14 miles driven.[29]

Surely, you've heard that it's important to reduce the use of fossil fuels by driving less— you know, ride your bike or walk instead or take public transportation. These are all helpful measures, but did you know that by taking animals off your plate you can also help curb emissions? "Animal agriculture is responsible for more annual CO_2 emissions than that produced by 400 million cars."[30] You know those semi-trucks you pass, carrying cattle or pigs to a slaughterhouse? Emitting CO_2. That ship or plane transporting meat halfway around the world to be sold? Emitting CO_2. Even that grass-fed, organic, cage-free meat had to be transported to wherever it is being sold.

27   Claire Schnaffnit-Chatterjee, "The Global Food Equation: Food Security in an Environment of Increasing Scarcity," Deutsche Bank Research, September 21, 2009, https://www.dbresearch.com.

28   "Sustainability SRJC," Santa Rosa Junior College, accessed February 25, 2022, https://sustainability.santarosa.edu/culture.

29   Suzy Amis Cameron, *The OMD Plan: Swap One Meal a Day to Save Your Health and Save the Planet* (New York: Simon & Schuster, 2019).

30   Joy, *Why We Love Dogs, Eat Pigs, and Wear Cows*, 77, 172; P. Gerber, H. Steinfeld, B. Henderson ,et al., *Tackling Climate Change Through Livestock: A Global Assessment of Emissions and Mitigation Opportunities* (Rome: FAO, 2013).

Learning how factory farms work and about their treatment of animals, as well as their effect on the environment around them (with sludge running into waterways and infecting drinking water, or their waste contributing to dead zones in the ocean) makes me think twice about the kinds of food I want to be eating and the kinds of industry I want to be supporting with my money.

So, whether you are changing your diet to avoid heart disease, diabetes, cancer, or a stroke, or you are changing your diet to help ensure planetary health for yourself and generations to come, you can rest assured you are making a difference with each bite you put in your mouth. How much of a difference? According to Stephanie Mantilla, "The estimated impact of eating meat every day costs one animal life, 1,100 gallons of water, 40 pounds of grain, 30 square feet of forest, and 20 pounds of CO_2. Every day you're a vegan saves the equivalent."[31]

I soon realized that not only was my body benefitting, but this lifestyle was making a difference in the health of the world. "Experts say that eliminating the consumption of animal products is the single greatest thing humans can do to alleviate climate change," says Anna Keeve with the T. Colin Campbell Center for Nutrition Studies.[32]

From time to time, our family enjoys eating plant-based No Evil brand's Italian sausage "meat." Their packaging states: "Imagine if every American left meat off their plate one day a week for one year. That'd be like taking 7.6 million cars off the

31   Stephanie Mantilla, "Vegan Calculator: What's The Environmental Impact of Going Vegan?" Plant Prosperous, November 16, 2021, https://plantprosperous.com/vegan-calculator.

32   Anna Keeve, "5 Climate Change Crisis Facts That Will Inspire Your Green Journey," T. Colin Campbell Center for Nutrition Studies, updated July 7, 2021, https://nutritionstudies.org/5-climate-change-crisis-facts-that-will-inspire-your-green-journey/.

road!" and "Bring back the road trip but don't forget the plant meat. Switching to a plant-based diet saves more carbon emissions than driving a hybrid. How much more? 50 percent more!" I feel good every time I open up one of their packages.

Any time you need motivation and wonder whether you can or should do this, you can think of all the water, grain, forests, CO_2 emissions and animals you are saving. You are giving yourself and the world a gift at the same time.

Our WFPBNO health journey begins

At the time we started on this journey, I thought, "How am I going to do this?" My kids were in early elementary school, ages six and eight, and money was tight. What if they weren't going to get what they needed for their growing bodies? What if nobody wanted to eat healthier foods? What if our friends and family thought we were crazy?

I realize the challenge of changing a family's eating habits may sound ambitious; with toddlers or elementary school age children in tow, just fitting in a shower and getting dressed can be challenging enough, not to mention making time for work, fun, and the hundreds of other responsibilities we have. But it's doable. Our family and many others are proof.

What follows is the information I wish I'd had when we started our journey away from eating SAD. I choose to believe that when we know better, we do better. You have in your hands the information you need to make an informed decision for yourself and your family. It took our family 10 years to get to where we knew enough to realize that we could have adopted this lifestyle in 10 days. I'll share with you all that I learned on our family's journey, saving you from having to go through some of the mistakes we did.

If I showed you a 10-day adjustment in your lifestyle that would save you *10 years* of trial-and-error maintenance on your car and keep it running for 300,000 miles you'd be thrilled. Somehow, for many people, our car breaking down is more important than our bodies breaking down.

I'd like nothing more than for you and your family to be healthy. Plus, I'd like to save you from wasting time and money and—as a natural byproduct—help save the planet. My aim is to teach you what I learned, and show you some simple paths to making healthier choices.

This book is for you if...

Maybe you've tried a Beyond Burger, or are currently doing keto to try to gain health and lose weight. Maybe you've heard about plant-based eating and are wondering what the hype is all about. As a loving parent, you might be looking for the healthiest way of eating for your family. Every year, billions of dollars are spent on the "diet" industry. You might be wondering if this book is just another in the long line of trends in eating.

This is not a gimmicky diet book.

This book is for you if you're tired of wondering if you're feeding your kids a healthy enough diet. You are in the right place if you are busy, have plenty of other things going on, and don't want to spend hours each day in the kitchen. It's for you if you have family members with health issues you'd like to avoid.

It's also for you if you're confused by all the "diet" information out there and want to know enough to make good choices but don't want to read books and more books on the subject or to research every new eating trend that comes along (paleo, keto, low-carb, Atkins, South Beach, juicing, intermittent fasting, gluten-free, etc.).

With the information in this book, you'll be confident you're giving your family all the nutrition they need to grow healthy and strong, you'll have more energy than you've had in years, and you'll save money in the process.

Why should I listen to you?

Like you, I love my family. Also, possibly like you, my family of origin has a history of heart disease, cancer, and diabetes. I've always been a problem solver and rigorous researcher so I sought solutions. I read books and articles and watched documentaries on plant-based eating. I earned my Plant-Based Nutrition Certificate from the T. Colin Campbell Center for Nutritional Studies (CNS) and eCornell. I completed a 12-Day McDougall program online. (The footnotes and citations are there for those of you who want to dig deeper, and substantiate the vast amount of research I waded through.) I taught a university-level nutrition class, and led corporate mindfulness and meditation workshops for one of the largest brokerage firms in the world. I'm certified in a neurological technique to help people get out of pain, as well as massage, yoga, Pilates and spiritual direction. I hold a Bachelor of Arts degree in Geography from the University of Washington.

I brought my family along for the ride (sometimes willingly, sometimes not so much), and learned a lot about how to integrate what I was learning into our full, active lives. Along the way, I've helped others make the transition.

I want you to feel the best you ever have and to rest in the confidence that you are doing all you can for your family and the planet by learning to eat differently.

The journey we take together

The outline below tracks the journey you'll be taking over the next week and a half. While 10 days may seem too quick for a lifestyle change, I assure you it's not. By following along, at the end of 10 days you'll be well on your way to making this new way of eating your everyday normal. We'll break it down day by day with the information you need, suggestions to try, and pitfalls to avoid. And if you're a parent like me, you will also find useful tips in this book that will help you transition your family from a SAD to a **H**ealthy **A**nd **P**lant **P**owered **Y**ay! (HAPPY) way of eating. (Since WFPBNO is a bit of a mouthful, I'll use it and HAPPY interchangeably.) Look for specific actions you can take at the end of each day.

On Day 1 you will learn what eating plant-based actually entails and why it makes such good sense for everybody on the planet (young and old).

Day 2 I will teach you how to make a successful and lasting start to a WFPBNO/HAPPY way of eating.

On Day 3 we'll discuss easy replacements and simple ways to prepare healthy foods that your family already enjoys eating.

On Day 4 I'll break down how to get those foods and simple

shopping tips. We'll also look at transition foods and their place in the process.

Day 5 we'll examine some common pitfalls and how to avoid them.

Day 6 we'll look at some simple and easy additions and subtractions to help you in your transition away from a SAD to better health for your family.

On Day 7 we'll cover pleasing kids, including how to get picky eaters on board and how to survive shocked parents and friends.

Days 8 and 9 we'll look at eating out and how to respond when people ask what you're doing and why.

And finally, on Day 10 we'll end with ways to stay encouraged to help you maintain your healthy new lifestyle.

With some simple and easy steps, you'll be transitioning away from a SAD to better health for your family. You'll be adopting the WFPBNO lifestyle. WFPBNO doesn't exactly roll off the tongue, does it? It leaves a lot to be desired but an easy way to think of it is you're going from…

SAD (Standard American Diet)
to HAPPY (Healthy And Plant-Powered, Yay!)

Now, let's get HAPPY!

DAY 1

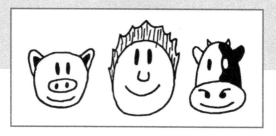

WHAT YOU NEED TO UNDERSTAND IN ORDER TO START AND SUCCEED

ON THIS FIRST day, let's get you up to speed on the facts and terminology so you know why this is so important. We'll start with some questions and answers.

WHY DON'T YOU SAY "VEGAN" INSTEAD OF "HAPPY" OR "WFPBNO?"

What do you picture in your mind when you hear the word "vegan?" A long-haired, patchouli oil scented, sandal wearing hippy who won't use honey and drives a Prius or old VW bus? No offense to any of those things (I have patchouli oil and used to drive an '87 Vanagon).

For a lot of people, the associations that come up with the word "vegan" are more related to social issues around what they eat than what they actually eat. Not to mention the fact that you could eat French fries, deep-fat fried tofu burgers, and Oreos at every meal and be vegan. And, of course, when I say vegan or WFPBNO, I think HAPPY! (Healthy And Plant-Powered, Yay!)

WAIT, I THOUGHT OLIVE/COCONUT/ AVOCADO OIL WERE GOOD FOR YOU?

We're attempting to eat real, whole plant foods in as unprocessed a way as possible without adding oil. Not because we have anything against vegetable oils except that, as T. Colin Campbell says, polyunsaturated fats (found in plants), "are susceptible to tissue damaging oxidation...Oxidation brings into consideration the formation of chemically reactive oxygen that *causes aging and increases cardiovascular disease and cancer.* For example, *plant oils experimentally promote cancer much more than saturated fats*—that's right (emphasis added). This is an experimental observation that is at least 30 to 40 years old."[33]

For those who have heard or read about the benefits of a Mediterranean diet, this one can be hard (Mom, I'm looking at you). Yes, the Mediterranean diet has health benefits, but that has more to do with the fact that it has more plant-based products and less animal products than the typical SAD diet. From a physiological standpoint, oil injures your endothelial cells, which line your blood vessels. These cells prevent adhesion and act as a barrier between blood and the rest of your body tissue. Healthy endothelial cells keep things flowing and prevent plaque build-up. Remember that plaque build-up

---

33   T. Colin Campbell, "Plant Oils Are Not a Healthy Alternative to Saturated Fat," T. Colin Campbell Center for Nutrition Studies, updated July 21, 2016, https://nutritionstudies.org/plant-oils-are-not-a-healthy-alternative-to-saturated-fat/.

can lead to clots blocking arteries—otherwise known as heart attacks.[34]

We all need some fat to stay healthy. A typical WFPBNO/ HAPPY diet provides 10 to 12 percent fat (coming from nuts, seeds, avocados, and vegetables). This is in comparison with a SAD diet, which is typically comprised of 30 to 50 percent fat from animals and oils. (One tablespoon of olive oil is the oil from 50 olives.[35] Could you eat 50 olives at one sitting? Can you easily use more than one tablespoon of olive oil at one sitting?) We don't pour oil down our sinks because it clogs the pipes. Similarly, when we pour oil into our bodies, it stiffens our arteries and impairs the ability of our arteries to dilate. Hamburgers, fries and cheesecake do this to our arteries. But so do olive, soybean and palm oils.[36]

At first, I couldn't comprehend how I was going to cook without oil. What about vegetable stir fry? Or roasted vegetables? And how about baking? Turns out, you can still make all these things— without oil. The easiest substitute for oil in cooking is water or broth. Where you'd add oil to fry, add water or broth. Or mix it up and try some soy sauce, or Worcestershire sauce, or even sherry or white wine. Roasting veggies? Same thing, instead of drizzling oil on top I use broth and herbs.

Baking is easy as well. Swap equal parts applesauce for the oil. Or use mashed banana. Your cakes, muffins, and cookies will still

---

34   "Olive Oil Injures Endothelial Cells," Whole Food Plant Based Diet, accessed February 25, 2022, https://www.wholefoodplantbaseddiet.com/olive-oil-injures-endothelial-cells/.

35   Rosemary Black, "How Many Olives are in 1 Tbsp of Olive Oil?" Parade, September 14, 2011, https://parade.com/111535/rosemaryblack/14-green-vs-black-olives/.

36   Oliveira, Rosane, "Is Olive Oil Bad for Your Heart?" Forks Over Knives, February 14, 2018. https://www.forksoverknives.com/wellness/why-olive-oil-is-not-healthy-for-your-heart/

be moist but without the extra fat you and your endothelial cells don't need.

One of the biggest boosts to your endothelial cells is nitric oxide. Nitric oxide is a vasodilator (a molecule produced naturally by your body that causes your blood vessels to dilate rather than constrict).[37] Where do you get nitric oxide? When you chew nitrates, they mix with bacteria in your mouth to produce nitric oxide. So, eat foods high in natural nitrates such as arugula, kale, Swiss chard, spinach, beet greens, bok choy, collard greens, mustard greens, asparagus, Brussels sprouts, Napa cabbage, broccoli, and cilantro.[38, 39]

By the way, vasodilation doesn't just help with blood flow in the heart. Eating greens can help with your love life as well. We're talking whole body HAPPY. Erectile dysfunction has been called a canary in the coalmine, since it can be a sign of blocked blood flow or hardening of the arteries.[40]

ISN'T EATING THIS WAY MORE EXPENSIVE?

This is a common misconception. The fact is, the opposite is actually true. I found I was actually saving money on groceries by buying whole plant-based foods. It turns out that when you take the meat, milk, cheese, yogurt, and ice cream out of your cart, you

37   Arlene Levine, David Punihaole, T. Barry Levine, "Characterization of the Role of Nitric Oxide and its Clinical Applications," *Cardiology* 122, no. 1 (2012): 55-68, https://pubmed.ncbi.nlm.nih.gov/22722323/.

38   Lindsay Boyers, "Fruits and Vegetables That Are High in Nitrates," Livestrong, updated November 18, 2019, https://www.livestrong.com/article/541308-fruits-vegetables-that-are-high-in-nitrates/.

39   "6 Foods to Send Nitric Oxide Levels Soaring," Touchstone Essentials, accessed February 25, 2022, https://thegoodinside.com/6-foods-to-send-nitric-oxide-levels-soaring/.

40   "Diet Away Erectile Dysfunction," Physicians Committee for Responsible Medicine, April 16, 2015, https://www.pcrm.org/news/blog/diet-away-erectile-dysfunction.

can literally fill it with grains, beans, lentils, fresh fruits, and veggies and still come out ahead.

If you're swapping out the foods you used to buy and replacing them with vegan processed foods (let's say swapping ice cream for coconut/soy/cashew ice cream or swapping hamburger for vegan "meat" crumbles) then you may find your grocery bill is only slightly different. We'll talk later about why we don't want to be eating these vegan processed products regularly and how to use them as transition foods on your journey if you choose to.

A five-pound bag of potatoes costs between $2.00 and $4.00 (depending on the type of potato and where you live).[41] You can make a wide variety of HAPPY dishes from a bag of potatoes. How about:

- Scalloped potatoes
- Hashed browns
- Mashed potatoes
- Baked potatoes
- Oven fries
- Potato wedges
- Potato skins
- Potato soup
- Potato tacos
- Potato curry
- Potato casserole
- Potato frittatas
- Potato salad
- Or my new favorite: potato waffles.

---

41   "How Much Do Potatoes Cost?" The Cold Wire, accessed February 25, 2022, https://www.thecoldwire.com/how-much-do-potatoes-cost/.

By comparison, a bag of chips will set you back $2.00 to $5.00, and won't provide near the nutritional value or meal option variety—not to mention the fact, if you're like me, they'll leave you hungry for more.[42]

WHAT DO YOU EAT IF YOU CAN'T EAT MEAT, CHEESE, OR EGGS? WHAT ELSE IS THERE?

Short answer: anything that doesn't have a mother, or a face. We eat fruits, vegetables, legumes (beans), nuts, grains, seeds. Most people get tripped up here because they can't imagine a meal without meat or dairy. After all, meat and dairy usually form the basis of a SAD meal.

Most people haven't had vegan lasagna, or black bean enchiladas. They've never tried a homemade veggie burger or plant-based meatloaf. They can't picture WFPBNO/HAPPY mashed potatoes and mushroom gravy. And they can't imagine vegetables and starches and carbohydrates making up the bulk of any given meal. This makes a certain amount of sense, because we all have a hard time envisioning things we haven't seen or tried.

It might help to remember that some of the biggest animals on the planet also eat this way. Elephants and rhinos eat WFPBNO/HAPPY.

I'M AN ENDURANCE ATHLETE, WILL I HAVE ENOUGH ENERGY?

---

42 "How Much Do Potato Chips Cost?" How Much Is It, August 14, 2018, https://www.howmuchisit.org/how-much-potato-chips-cost/.

If Scott Jurek (an ultra-marathoner) can win races of a hundred miles or more eating a plant-based diet, then I think it'll be all right for you.[43]

Pro NBA star Kyrie Irving says going plant-based has made him a stronger player.[44] MMA and former UFC fighter James Wilks went vegan after sustaining an injury.[45] Pro cyclist Dotsie Bausch went vegan in 2009 and went on to win a silver medal at the 2012 Olympics.[46] Seven-time Formula One champion Lewis Hamilton went vegan in 2017.[47] Plant-based surfer Tia Blanco won back-to-back gold medals in 2015 and 2016.[48]

Canadian figure skater Meagan Duhamel, with three Olympic medals to her name, wrote on her blog, Lutz of Greens, "It's simply healthier. Vegans eat more fiber, fruits, and vegetables, therefore getting more vitamins and minerals into their bodies. Vegans also don't eat saturated fat and their protein comes from clean sources, free of antibiotics and chemicals."[49]

Colin Kaepernick. Olympic weightlifter Kendrick Farris. Australian Olympic sprinter Morgan Mitchell. Pro NFL linebacker Derrick Morgan. All these professional athletes have made the switch. U.S. women's soccer star Alex Morgan. Professional basketball players DeAndre Jordan and Javale McGee. The list goes on and on.[50]

---

43   Luke Darby, "The Real-Life Diet of the Vegan Who Can Run Hundreds of Miles, No Problem," *GQ*, October 13, 2015, https://www.gq.com/story/the-real-life-diet-of-the-ultramarathoner-who-gave-up-meat-and-became-vegan.

44   Jill Ettinger, "NBA Star Kyrie Irving Says a Vegan Diet is Making Him a Stronger Player," Live Kindly, accessed February 25, 2022, https://www.livekindly.co/global-meat-invest-vegan-protein/.

45   Audrey Enjoli, "19 Vegan Athletes Who Swear by Plant-Based Diets," Live Kindly, accessed February 25, 2022, https://www.livekindly.co/vegan-athletes-swear-by-plants.

46   Ibid.

47   Ibid.

48   Ibid.

49   Ibid.

50   Ibid.

Okay, so now you know a bit more about this whole food plant-based approach to eating. Next, we'll explore what HAPPY/ WFPBNO can do specifically for you, your health, your wallet and the planet.

Learning what WFPBNO/HAPPY can do

> "The most violent weapon on
> earth is the table fork."
> —Unknown

Health benefits in real terms

> "There are only two kinds of cardiologists:
> those who are vegan and those
> who haven't read the data."
> —Dr. Kim Williams, past-president of the
> American College of Cardiology.[51]

The benefits of eating HAPPY are many. Preventing and re-versing heart disease (our number one killer in the U.S.) seems like it should be reason enough. May I ask, has anyone in your family had a heart attack or a stroke? Or does anyone have high blood pressure or diabetes? These conditions can be prevented— and often even reversed—by dietary and lifestyle changes. Is there a history of cancer in your family? It has been shown that what you eat—specifically plant protein instead of animal protein (casein)—can prevent or stop the growth of cancer cells.[52]

Do you or someone you know have to take insulin to deal

---

51   Rich Roll, interview with Dr. Kim Williams, podcast audio, November 5, 2017,
      https://www.richroll.com/podcast/kim-williams/.
52   Mayo Clinic Staff, "Nutrition and Healthy Eating," Mayo Clinic, October 30,
      2019, https://www.mayoclinic.org/healthy-lifestyle/nutrition-and-healthy-eating/
      in-depth/how-plant-based-food-helps-fight-cancer/art-20457590.

with type 2 diabetes? With a third of the American population obese,[53] and diabetes being the eighth leading cause of death in the U.S.,[54] this problem is growing. But even diabetes can be helped and, in many cases, reversed once people change to a high carbohydrate, low fat, high fiber diet instead of the SAD. Many people have gotten off insulin within three weeks[55] of changing to a WFPBNO diet. [56, 57] Other byproducts of WFPBNO include: preventing strokes, increasing overall health, stamina, blood flow, and let's not forget decreasing excess weight, just to name a few.

In the United States, someone has a heart attack every 40 seconds.[58] On his Facebook page, Rip Esselstyn, author of *My Beef with Meat*[59] and *The Engine 2 Diet* recalls:[60] "Over the course of my dozen years with the Austin Fire Department, my crew responded to more than 50 heart attacks—we were only able to resuscitate three patients. Three!" Wouldn't you like to reduce your

53 "Overweight and Obesity Statistics," National Institute of Diabetes and Digestive and Kidney Diseases, updated September 2021, https://www.niddk.nih.gov/health-information/health-statistics/overweight-obesity.

54 "Deaths and Mortality," Centers for Disease Control and Prevention, updated January 13, 2022, https://www.cdc.gov/nchs/fastats/leading-causes-of-death.htm.

55 Neal Barnard. "Diabetes." Physicians Committee for Responsible Medicine, 2022. https://www.pcrm.org/health-topics/diabetes.

56 John McDougall, "Dr. McDougall's Response to: Looking Past Blood Sugar to Survive With Diabetes by Gina Kolata in the August 20, 2007 *New York Times,*" The McDougall Newsletter, August 2007, https://www.drmcdougall.com/misc/2007nl/aug/nyt.pdf.

57 "Diabetes," Physicians Committee for Responsible Medicine, accessed February 25, 2022, https://www.pcrm.org/health-topics/diabetes.

58 "Heart Disease Facts," Centers for Disease Control and Prevention, updated February 7, 2022, https://www.cdc.gov/heartdisease/facts.htm.

59 Rip Esselstyn, *My Beef with Meat: The Healthiest Argument for Eating a Plant-strong Diet* (New York: Grand Central Life & Style, 2013).

60 Rip Esselstyn, "In the United States, someone has a heart attack every 40 seconds. (cdc.gov) Over the course of my dozen years with the Austin Fire Department, my crew responded to more than 50 heart attacks—we were only able to resuscitate three patients. Three…" Facebook, February 14, 2021, https://www.facebook.com/RipEsselstyn/photos/in-the-united-states-someone-has-a-heart-attack-every-40-seconds-cdcgov-over-the/1070904310089944/.

chance of having a heart attack?

Who among us doesn't know someone affected by breast cancer? American breast cancer surgeon, Dr. Kristi Funk, known for her surgical treatment of celebrities Angelina Jolie and Sheryl Crow[61] says, "Breast cancer is one of the most feared diseases in the world. But did you know that only five to 10 percent of all breast cancer comes from an inherited gene mutation? That's right: Up to 90 percent of cancer results from the dietary and lifestyle choices we make every single day—not genetics."[62]

The Physicians Committee for Responsible Medicine recently reported, "Men who consume the most plant-based foods decrease their risk of dying from prostate cancer by 19 percent, according to an abstract published in *The Journal of Urology*. Researchers compared plant-based diet intake and prostate cancer incidence and mortality rates for 47,243 men as part of the Health Professionals Follow-Up Study. Adherence to a plant-based diet lowered the risk of death from cancer as well as risk for total and advanced cancer among younger men. These results show the efficacy of plant-based diets for cancer prevention and survival."[63]

Forks Over Knives posted on Twitter, "Research shows that moving to a whole-food, plant-based diet can reduce the symptoms of

61   Murray Scougall, "Surgeon to the Stars Says Rates of Breast Cancer Could Reduce if Women Helped Themselves Dodge Disease," *The Sunday Post,* July 23, 2018, https://www.sundaypost.com/fp/of-course-you-can-do-all-the-right-things-and-still-get-it-but-we-have-a-lot-of-power-over-this-we-should-use-it/.

62   Courtney Davison, "'It's Empowering': Surgeon Kristi Funk on Diet and Reducing Breast Cancer Risk," Forks Over Knives, updated September 27, 2021, https://www.forksoverknives.com/wellness/surgeon-kristi-funk-diet-reducing-breast-cancer-risk/.

63   "Plant-Based Diets Decrease Risk of Death from Prostate Cancer," Physicians Committee for Responsible Medicine, September 24, 2021, https://www.pcrm.org/news/health-nutrition/plant-based-diets-decrease-risk-death-prostate-cancer.

type 1 diabetes and can help manage and even reverse type 2 diabetes and prediabetes."[64] Managing diabetes, or your child's diabetes is a serious job. Isn't it one you'd like to not have to worry about? "Through lifestyle changes, you may be able to achieve a complete remission of type 2 diabetes, even if you've been suffering with the disease for decades. In fact, you can start improving your health within a matter of hours,"[65] says Dr. Michael Greger, author of *How Not To Die.*

NutritionFacts.org posted on Facebook, "When the World Health Organization designated bacon, ham, hot dogs, lunch meat, and sausage to be Group 1 carcinogens, meaning we know these products cause cancer in human beings, who cares if it's the heme iron, the heterocyclic aromatic amines, the polycyclic aromatic hydrocarbons or the N-nitrosamines? They're all wrapped up in the same place—processed meat—which we know causes cancer. The landmark Global Burden of Disease Study found that processed meats are to be blamed for the deaths of more than 800,000 people every year. The NIH-AARP study of more than 500,000 Americans suggested that 20 percent of heart disease deaths among American women could be averted if the highest consumers of processed meat would cut down to the equivalent of less than a half strip of bacon a day."[66]

It's facts like those that helped me steer the grocery cart away

64   Forks Over Knives (@forksoverknives), "Research shows that moving to a whole-food, plant-based diet can reduce the symptoms of type 1 diabetes and can help manage and even reverse type 2 diabetes and prediabetes. http://bit.ly/2LGkyND," Twitter post, July 9, 2019, 2:00 PM, https://twitter.com/ForksOverKnives/status/1148653050137075712?ref_src=twsrc%5Etfw.

65   Nutritionfacts.org, "We should stay away from processed meats, regardless of the mechanism by which they cause cancer. Every year, more than five million expected years of life are lost to lung cancer, breast cancer, and colorectal cancer alone…" Facebook post, October 12, 2021, https://www.facebook.com/NutritionFacts.org/photos/a.505323302817517/5105743022775499/?type=3&_rdr.

66   Michael Greger, "What About the Heme in Impossible Burgers?" NutritionFacts.org, February 15, 2021, https://nutritionfacts.org/video/what-about-the-heme-in-impossible-burgers/.

from the bacon and lunch meat my family wanted. I couldn't unlearn what I'd learned, and couldn't knowingly feed my family carcinogenic food.

Immune systems

"We should all be eating fruits and vegetables as if our lives depend on it—because they do."
—Dr. Michael Greger[67]

In August of 2021, Dr. Stephan Esser, MD posted on Instagram, "People tell me that 'healthy Americans' are dying every day from a viral illness. I ask them who are these "healthy Americans" when the CDC says that:

1:3 has high blood pressure

1:6 has high cholesterol

1:9 has type 2 diabetes

70% are overweight or obese

<23% get recommended daily exercise

9% get recommended daily veggie intake

12% get recommended daily fruit intake

50% of calories come from flour, oil, and sugar

Pediatric obesity has tripled

36 million smoke everyday

1:8 Americans fit criteria for alcohol disorder[68]

We are a sick, obese, overmedicated, under exercised, inadequately slept, substance abusing society. Until we look in the mirror

---

67   "664: Dr. Michael Greger and How Not to Diet, The Ultimate Weight Loss Guide," *The Healthification Podcast,* podcast, January 26, 2020, MP3 Audio, 35:03, https://strongbodygreenplanet.com/e664-dr-michael-greger-and-how-not-to-diet-the-ultimate-weight-loss-guide/.

68   @ Esserhealth, Instagram post, August 23, 2021, https://www.instagram.com/p/CS8CpUXDR7L/.

and admit this, there is no hope and people will continue to die prematurely of both common (heart disease, diabetes, hormonal cancers) and uncommon causes (MERS, H1N1, COVID)."[69]

In the last few years, you may have thought more about your immune system and how to help strengthen it. Nutrition consultant Theresa "Sam" Houghton says, "Your immune system is best prepared to take action again viruses when you choose foods that provide a steady stream of key nutrients. Diets centered around whole plant foods in particular appear to stimulate natural killer cell activity. Natural killer cells are part of the innate immune response that homes in on pathogens, including viruses responsible for common respiratory infections."[70]

Houghton continues, "We now know there are foods that weaken the immune system. Some foods hinder immune function, which can make you more susceptible to viral infection:

- Fried foods promote inflammation, which dampens overall immune response.
- Highly processed foods, including refined grains and sugars, deplete nutrients and prevent proper immune function.
- Meat may be a source of food-borne pathogens—including viruses—and toxic chemicals, both of which can interfere with your immune system. Many animal products have also been shown to increase inflammation.[71]

69   @Esserhealth, Instagram post, September 23, 2021, https://www.instagram.com/p/ CULTe2sLLTS/.

70   Theresa "Sam" Houghton, "How Does Nutrition Affect the Immune System?" T. Colin Campbell Center for Nutrition Studies, March 20, 2020, https:// nutritionstudies.org/how-does-nutrition-affect-the-immune-system/.

71   Ibid.

Even if you do everything you can and still catch something that is going around, studies are showing that plant-based eaters are faring better than those eating the Standard American Diet (SAD). In 2021 the British Medical Journal published a study concluding, "Plant-based eaters are 73% less likely to suffer moderate to severe COVID-19. A new study has revealed a link between diet and COVID-19, finding that plant-based eaters were 73% less likely to become severely ill from the virus compared with those who included animals in their diets, even after accounting for potentially confounding factors."[72]

It's not just your health that benefits, the world benefits as well

Remember those 106 gallons of water that *Business Insider* reported go into making an ounce of beef? They followed up that fact by saying, "By comparison, just about 23 gallons are needed for an ounce of almonds. So stop with the almond shaming, and start eating less red meat."[73]

There's discussion around the type of water being used to raise livestock. Is rainwater growing the grass that cattle need to eat? For part of their lives, maybe so, if they're lucky. But when they're in feedlots, where a blade of grass is not to be found, they are eating grain that was grown using crop irrigation, drinking water that may or may not be from a rain catchment system, and utilizing gray water to dilute their waste. And that's just beef. Pigs and chickens are almost solely raised in confinement in the U.S., thus requiring a lot of water.

---

72   "Plant-based and /or fish diets may help lessen severity of COVID-19 infection," BMJ, June 7, 2021, https://www.bmj.com/company/newsroom/plant-based-and -or-fish-diets-may-help-lessen-severity-of-covid-19-infection/.
73   Erin Brodwin, "One Chart Sums Up the Real Problem in the California Drought— and It Isn't Almonds," *Business Insider*, April 13, 2015, https://www.businessinsider. com/real-villain-in-the-california-drought-isnt-almonds--its-red-meat-2015-4.

In many parts of the world, access to clean water is an issue. Where I live, we've been under drought water restrictions for the past eight years. And yet it takes more than 2,400 gallons of water to produce just one pound of meat according to peta.org. So a quarter-pounder hamburger uses 600 gallons of water. For one burger.[74]

It's not just the water that's being used, it's the land as well. Vast swaths of the rain forests are being cut and burned for grazing cattle. To feed cattle and pigs worldwide, crops such as soy, alfalfa, and corn are being grown where forests once stood. These vast monoculture crops have an adverse effect on the biodiversity of an area, and require fossil fuels in the form of nitrogen along with pesticides to amend the soil when it becomes depleted. As we previously covered, these fertilizers and chemicals then run off fields and into streams, creeks, and rivers and eventually lead to dead zones in oceans.

According to a Plantstrong by Engine 2 post on Facebook, "Erosion destroys the ability of land to regenerate itself and eventually turns it into a lifeless desert. Farming is one of the leading causes of erosion in the U.S. with 90% of farmland losing soil at a rate 75 times greater than what's considered sustainable. Ranches and crop farms are both to blame, but erosion from plant farming happens at a rate six times slower than erosion from meat farming."[75]

Google "palm oil production" and "deforestation" and check out the pictures of the rain forest razed to produce palm oil.

74   "How Much Water Does It Take to Make One Steak?" PETA, accessed February 25, 2022, https://www.peta.org/videos/meat-wastes-water.

75   Plantstrong by Engine 2, Facebook post, April 22, 2020, https://www.facebook.com/GoPlantstrong/photos/a.424803913376/10158102271148377/?type=3&eid=ARD2FzDL0OZjGbYpy0GD1pj8owPI0Rmar2kic0a0kgRddOxC-qnQBG01aZp HufwgTc0SCkf42DXq7mIH.

Palm oil helps stabilize products such as snack and protein bars, candy, and chocolates. We lose 25 orangutans a day to deforestation.[76] Have you seen the commercial for peanut butter with the orangutan?[77] It's a good one to show your kids. Here again, we can vote with our dollars and not buy products that have artery clogging oil in them and whose production is neither good for us nor good for the planet.

If we're serious about wanting to do all we can to lessen our impact on global warming, then taking meat off our plates is something we can do that has an impact three times a day—breakfast, lunch, and dinner. We don't have to choose between our health and planetary health—by adopting a HAPPY way of eating, we are killing two birds with one stone. (Or more accurately, saving birds, pigs, cows, water, and air all at the same time).

As plant-based author Rip Esselstyn sums it up: "Why go plant-based? Average annual amount of CO_2 emitted from vegan diet: 1,055kg. Average annual amount of CO_2 emitted from diets of meat-eater: 2,055kg.[78] Vegans have a 32% decreased chance in developing heart disease and a 23% decreased chance in developing type 2 diabetes. Impact of livestock industry: 30% of national water footprint in the US alone, 14.5% of global greenhouse gasses produced, 45% of global land is occupied by livestock."[79]

76   Karen Rockett, "Orangutan Population Falls by 25 Every Day—And Food We
      Eat Is to Blame," the *Mirror*, August 17, 2019, https://www.mirror.co.uk/news/
      uk-news/orangutan-population-falls-25-every-18952462.
77   Rainforest Action Network, "AMAZING! Orangutan Asks Girl for Help in Sign
      Language," YouTube video, 2:21, October 9, 2013, https://www.youtube.com/
      watch?v=G32YehcdUAw.
78   Nicole Axworthy. "Meat-Eaters Produce Nearly 60 Percent More Greenhouse Gases
      than Vegetarians, Study Finds." VegNews.com, December 3, 2021. https://vegnews.
      com/2021/12/meat-eaters-greenhouse-gases-vegetarians.
79   Plantstrong by Engine 2.

We're attempting a 10-day challenge to change the way we eat. But even just a week of eating plant-based can have a major impact on our personal health and the impact we have on our planet.

As Dr. Caldwell B. Esselstyn Jr. put it, "According to @physicianscommittee "a plant-based diet can help reduce greenhouse gases, preserve water and land, and save lives." Eating a plant-based diet could be the "single biggest way" to reduce your environmental impact on earth. A plant-based diet could reduce one's carbon footprint from food up to 73%. Simply stated, a plant-based diet can improve and protect our own health and well-being, and that of Mother Earth."[80]

As Michael Greger explains, "What makes designing a sustainable diet so easy is that the same advice is good for personal health and planetary health. In California, including more animal products in your diet requires an additional 10,000 quarts of water a week. That's like taking 150 more showers each week. Instead of eating meat every day, if you skip meat on weekdays, you could conserve thousands of gallons of water a week and cut your daily carbon footprint and total ecological footprint by about 40 percent. What's more, replacing animal products with plant-based foods could reduce greenhouse gas emissions by up to 84 percent."

As the world population grows, and more people in more countries can afford to eat animal products, the demand for meat will only continue to rise. (This is a worldwide trend—rise above poverty and start eating more of a SAD.) Already, companies are

---

80 NutritionFacts.org, "Which Foods Have the Lowest Carbon Footprint?" YouTube video, 5:34, November 16, 2020, https://www.youtube.com/watch?v=IWKCvP1XCjA.

growing chicken and beef in labs, trying to find cost-effective and creative ways to meet demand without having to waste resources on the actual bird or animal. While this meat helps lessen animal and environmental cruelty, it is still meat and will affect your health negatively. It also costs $50 to make a single chicken nugget right now.[81]

If your only reason to eat HAPPY/WFPBNO is to reduce animal cruelty, these arguments may sound good to you. If, however, you're looking to lower cholesterol, avoid heart disease, avoid type 2 diabetes, lower blood pressure, and feel better, I'd treat them like the animal product they are and avoid them.

Looking at a world projected to reach 12 billion people, with a growing number of people moving into middle class and able to afford more of a SAD way of eating has driven me to look at sustainability in a new way. Learning about so-called "urban deserts," or the more recently coined phrase "food apartheids," where there are no grocery stores in low-income areas (primarily affecting people of color), makes me think about food equity and what I can do about it. I now support those who grow food, food cooperatives, and farm-to-school programs.

On a larger scale, I've written and called my politicians asking for changes in the Food Bill and for changes in how money is allocated in farming practices. I'm continuing to learn about zoning and how it impacts where grocery stores and fast-food restaurants can be—and why.

---

81   Deena Shanker, "These $50 Chicken Nuggets Were Grown in a Lab," Bloomberg, October 22, 2019, https://www.bloomberg.com/news/articles/2019-10-22/clean-meat-just-chicken-nuggets-grown-in-a-lab-coming-soon.

Finding your HAPPY "why" for changing how you eat (or, linking your heart with your head)

I really do believe that, for the most part, when we as people know better, we choose to do better. What do you know now that you want to change? I personally want to be able to look my grandkids in the eyes and tell them I did everything I could to be part of the solution when it came to climate change, not to mention their health.

Finding your own "why" for making a change is important. That why may change over time, but knowing what it is that propels you forward will help when someone asks why you're choosing to do what you're doing. It will also help when you feel like buying the ice cream or chicken nuggets for your kids when they're begging for them.

Are you concerned about your—or your child's—health? Are you concerned about the planet's health? Or maybe you want to reduce what you spend on food. Whatever your reason(s), have them at the forefront of your mind.

A note here about starting out. Knowing yourself can help you be successful when you start out in something unfamiliar. Are you someone who likes to dive in head first and not look back until you've completed what you set out to do? Are you someone who sees things very black and white? Or are you someone who likes to wade in slowly, gathering information and making small changes when they feel doable or only when you know you'll be able to be successful? There is no one right way to make a change, and the goal here is not perfection. The goal is to understand why you want to make the change and to embark on the journey, knowing there will be ups and downs and that you have everything at your disposal to make good decisions going forward.

By nature, I tend to be a black and white person (I'm a recovering perfectionist), and years of beating myself up after slipping backwards didn't help my movement forward. It took me a long time to learn to quickly change course after a mistake. For instance, I'd wake up ready to make good eating decisions. I'd have my coffee black without anything added to it (a win!), have some fruit, and a bowl of cereal, and then, say, meet a friend for lunch. If I decided to indulge in some chips (my Achilles' heel) with my sandwich, well then, the day was over.

I'd ruined my perfect day of eating and now in my mind it was all downhill anyway, so I might as well have pizza for dinner and ice cream for dessert and start all over with a clean slate tomorrow. Sound familiar to anyone? This was me for years. Thankfully, I'm much kinder to myself now. I think differently about what I'm eating, and if I really want something I'll have it, without the self-imposed guilt trip afterward. And, if I regret it, I choose to let it go and start again right then and there, not the next morning, (or the next week, or next January).

Consider how you tend to do things

Expect making this eating change to be similar to the way you approach other things, unless you're actively deciding to go about it differently. If you're someone who likes to gather information and take small steps, then adding one WFPBNO/HAPPY food option to a meal for a week or taking away a SAD food from a meal for a week may work better for you than purging your kitchen and pantry of all the foods you plan on eliminating.

On the other hand, maybe you're fully convinced that you need to make this change for health reasons and don't want any tempting foods around. In that case, getting rid of things you don't want to eat might be a great option to help you in your process of moving forward. The bottom line is that there is freedom here to work with yourself rather than against yourself. Once you know your "why," trust your instinct and start with whatever step feels attainable.

Lastly, if you're making this change for health reasons, I highly recommend scheduling a blood draw to have your lipid panel done for a benchmark. You can tell your doctor what you're doing and ask for a second blood draw 10 days later to compare. This may be covered by your insurance, or you may have to pay out of pocket, but it will be well worth the money. While you're doing the hard work of changing what you're putting into your mouth and body, it might feel like not much is happening since you can't *feel* your cholesterol or blood pressure dropping—among the other changes that are occurring. Having the bloodwork to prove what's working will reinforce your behavior and likely surprise your doctor (in a good way).

You're never too old to learn new ways of being. New York City's first vegan mayor, Eric Adams, says, "My mother joined me in eating plant-based at 80 years old. Fifteen years as a diabetic. Seven years on insulin. After two months whole-food plant-based, she threw her insulin away."[82] If 80-year-olds can change the way they eat and reverse disease, surely we can too.

Have you ever thought, "Gosh, I'd love to try that new restaurant in town that I've been hearing about," or, "I wish I had

---

82 Physicians Committee for Responsible Medicine, Facebook post, November 4, 2021, https://fb.watch/bvPlIkqLrm/.

the courage to try something I've never tried before." Maybe you've been on a trip and tried exotic local dishes in a foreign land. WFPBNO/HAPPY can be just as fun and exciting. This is not a destination, but rather a journey to places you've never been to before and to things you've never experienced. Let's use your "why" to get HAPPY. You've already learned a lot, now let's put that knowledge into action—no passport necessary for this journey! Next up, we'll look at exactly how to transition from SAD to HAPPY.

For fork's sake, LET'S DO THIS!

- Watch *Forks Over Knives* or *Gamechangers*.
- Extra time or love to read? Order *The China Study*.
- Look up the video on orangutans and palm oil: https://youtu.be/TQQXstNh45g.
- Watch Melanie Joy's TEDTalk: "Toward Rational, Authentic Food Choices."[83]
- Want to watch your cholesterol drop? Schedule a blood draw before you start and one 10 days later.

83　TEDx Talks, "Toward Rational, Authentic Food Choices | Melanie Joy | TEDxMünchen," YouTube video, February 5, 2015, https://www.youtube.com/watch?v=o0VrZPBskpg.

DAY 2

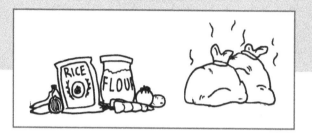

START NOW! YOU HAVE EVERYTHING YOU NEED TO START TODAY!

IT'S TIME FOR the Great Clean Out. You will Marie Kondo your kitchen, my friend. It's not possible to go full WFPBNO/HAPPY without getting rid of the offending foods. Removing temptation is a proven strategy. When an alcoholic decides to quit drinking, should they keep three cans from the six-pack of beer in the refrigerator just in case they get thirsty? Or hang on to a bottle of Scotch for a special occasion? Of course not.

It's hard to eat things you don't have, but easy to eat tempting treats you hid from yourself. (While your taste buds will change, your memory of where you hid the secret candy stash won't.) In my family, when we started out we got rid of everything we didn't want to eat, except things we'd use in moderation (chocolate chips, for instance). But then, on many evenings after putting the kids to bed—somewhere between 8:30 and 9:00 p.m.—I'd find my husband with a small bowl of chocolate chips in hand. I'd do my best to not chide him, and kept my distance so as not to cave in myself. Eventually, I stopped keeping chocolate chips on hand for a while, so it would not be a tempting late-night snack.

It might feel drastic to get rid of everything, but as Dr. Caldwell Esselstyn says in the documentary, *Forks Over Knives,* "Some people think the plant-based, whole-foods diet is extreme. Half a million people a year will have their chests opened up and a vein taken from their leg and sewn onto their coronary artery. Some people would call that extreme."

You can choose—through many small decisions—the future that Dr. Esselstyn was describing above (commonly known as by-pass surgery), or choose instead to benefit your body in so many ways along with your wallet and our planet. We're really just picking the kind of "extreme" we choose to deal with here.

My goal is to show you the quick-start method, the one where it doesn't take years and years to make changes. You don't have to have willpower made of steel here—we're attempting to make this as easy as possible.

Where to actually start. What to keep and what to toss.

How exactly do you do the Great Clean Out? You toss it.

Do I mean the good, really expensive dipping olive oil? Yes, I do. The olive tapenade packed with oil? Yes. The crackers, cookies, chips, white bread, ice cream, cheese, meat? Yes, all of it. If it makes you feel better, you can give it to someone who will use it (though knowing what you know now from Day 1, that might not feel very altruistic).

While it may initially be painful to toss those Parmesan crisp chips, that cottage cheese, or the store-bought cookies, the joy you will feel from eating what your body needs will outweigh the angst you feel in letting them go. (As a bonus, you may be able to see the back of your refrigerator or cupboard for the first time in a long time.) This is where your knowledge from Day 1 is going to pay off. You now know what whole foods are. You know what plant-based means, and soon you'll be able to identify hidden oils in food.

Let's start with the refrigerator. Any food that comes from an animal should go. All meat, dairy, cheese, milk, eggs, and ice cream. Remember things like yogurt, coffee creamer, salad dressings, and butter. If it didn't come from an animal, or doesn't have a mother, then leave it in the fridge.

After the refrigerator is cleaned out, move on to the cupboards. Here we're looking to get rid of food products that have oil, and/or animal products in them. When looking at processed food (or something that started out as a whole, plant-based food that then was mixed, added to, and packaged...I'm looking at you, fresh potatoes and corn, that end up becoming Doritos) see if you can read the ingredients.

You may be surprised by what and how many different ingredients can be in as simple a food item as crackers, or salad dressing. Some suggest a "five ingredients or less" rule. I'd suggest at least being able to pronounce the ingredients you plan on eating, or at the *very* least knowing what they are.

Keep all those whole grains you currently have. I'm talking flour, rice, quinoa, oatmeal, pasta, polenta, oil-free tortillas, pitas and lavash, whole grain bread. These, along with some potatoes can be the bases of almost all your meals. While digging through the cupboards, make sure you have some legumes or beans on hand, these can be black, pinto, kidney, cannellini, garbanzo, lentils—whatever type you and your family already like. Whether they are dried or canned doesn't matter, just have some on hand to get you going.

You may be looking around at what is left wondering just what it is you'll be eating. But don't worry, you'll have lots of options. You don't have to rush out and spend a lot of money on vegan replacements (we'll get to those later). The next time you're at the store you can look for crackers without oil and plant-based milk and yogurt.

But I'm going to miss all that food!

Maybe you think you can skip this step, or ease into going HAPPY or WFPBNO. If that's the way you want to do it, then go for it. If you want to make just a 10% change in your diet, say, cutting out meat one day a week to start, then that's great! Just remember that you will only be getting 10% of the benefit of this way of eating. I'm not saying that any small changes aren't worth doing—they are, and any changes you can make will help in the long run.

I was talking to a friend on the phone recently and she said, "Don't take this wrong, but I don't know how you can eat what you do. I don't like any of those foods!" Don't panic when looking at what food you have left. At first glance, you might not be excited about eating those dried lentils you had on hand in case of an emergency, but guess what, your tastes are going to change, and rapidly (more on this later). Plus, you'll be introducing all sorts of new options, so remind yourself of all the things you *can* have rather than dwelling on what you are choosing not to have.

What to do with what I have left?

Take stock of what you have that is WFPBNO/HAPPY in your possession. We're going to start by using it. Do you have a starch (rice, potatoes, quinoa, pasta)? Start there. This could mean cooking up a big pot (or rice cooker or Insta-Pot) of whatever you have on hand. Or, if you're short on time, maybe it's microwaving a pouch of rice or some potatoes, or cooking some pasta. The key here is to use what you have and make a lot of it. You'll thank yourself later.

Next, grab some of those beans (or lentils) you found while cleaning out the cupboard. Do what you did with the grains and cook up a big batch of them. Dinner could be as simple as some rice and beans (add some sautéed onions, bell peppers, greens of any kind, or any other veggies you like and those rice and beans just turned fancy). Add a side of crunchy veggies or a salad and some fresh fruit and you just made an awesome WFPBNO/HAPPY meal.

"But wait, I'm not a cook, I hate to cook!" you say? Okay, then do like dietitian and nutritionist Jeff Novick did when he started eating this way as a single parent with a 10-year-old daughter who needed to be able to prepare the food as well. As he says, "All you need is a large pot, a spoon, scissors, and a can opener to make this soup. Now what could be easier than that?"

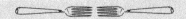

Jeff's Longevity Soup

7 cups water

15-oz can diced tomatoes

15-oz can crushed tomatoes

2 15-oz cans beans (whatever type you prefer)

2 pounds frozen vegetables (Italian blend or California blend
work well here, but so do carrots, peas, and corn mix)

2-3 cups of your favorite cooked starch (potatoes, grains, rice) or
½-1 cup uncooked pasta

Herbs/seasonings you like to taste (maybe Italian, or cumin,
paprika, and ginger)

Place all the ingredients into a pot and mix well. Bring to a boil
and simmer for 15 minutes until all vegetables are done.[84]

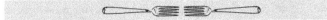

You're not going to have to cook like this every day. By cooking up big batches of rice/beans/pasta/quinoa, you are cooking
like a professional and utilizing the "batch cooking" method.
You'll use some of this food today, and some tomorrow and,
depending on how much you made or how you store it (frozen
beans work great later), you could be eating off this batch for a
week or more.

84　Jeff Novick, "Jeff's Longevity Soup," Dr. McDougall Health
　　& Medical Center, accessed February 25, 2022, https://www.
　　drmcdougall.com/recipes/jeffs-longevity-soup/.

There's nothing saying you have to eat or feed your family a fancy four-course dinner every night. It might be easiest for everyone if you simplify things and have bean burritos three times this week. Then again, maybe variety is the spice of your life and you have some time to kill and you're motivated to see what you can make using WFPBNO recipes you found online. You do you.

Help! What are we going to eat tonight?

Well, it depends on what you had left in your pantry, refrigerator, and cupboards, but let's say you cooked up a big batch of rice and beans. You could have that for dinner: a bowl of rice, topped with beans and your favorite salsa. Did you make a big pot of Jeff's Longevity soup? Enjoy that. Still hungry, have another bowl or two!

If you have some lettuce, you could make a big Southwest salad, adding some frozen or canned corn, tomatoes, maybe cilantro and green onion. Try tossing some of the rice and beans you cooked into the lettuce as well. Salsa could be your dressing, or you could always Google WFPBNO salad dressings and whip up one of those. (I learned the easiest dressing in the world from the McDougall program: equal parts maple syrup and mustard, add water to your desired thickness. Any mustard works.)

Have a little more time? How about homemade black bean burgers, using the beans and rice you cooked up?

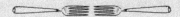

Take one can of beans (black or pinto work well here), drain them and mash them in a medium size bowl. To the beans, add:

1/4 cup of your cooked grain (rice or quinoa)
1/3 cup of oats
1 Tbsp of mustard
2 Tbsp ketchup
1 tsp of onion
1 tsp of garlic powder

Mix all ingredients* together, divide into four patties and bake at 400 degrees for seven minutes, flip and bake for seven minutes more.

Place those patties between slices of bread, or in a pita, or crumble them into a wrap, add whatever burger-type fixins' you like (lettuce, onion, tomato, pickles, mustard, and ketchup) and your easy WFPBNO dinner just went up a serious notch.

*(Chopped greens, corn, chopped bell pepper—you can add all kinds of veggies to these burger patties, so feel free to experiment and use whatever you have on hand).

Go to www.forforkssakebook.com for easy burger variations and ideas.

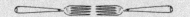

The goal is to cut out animal products and oil, not to suffer through 10 days of eating plain, bland food. You shouldn't be hungry at any point—there are plenty of great things to eat. It's about learning your preferences and figuring out what to have on hand for you and your family.

Remember that bowl of chocolate chips my husband had before going to bed? Over time, that bowl of chocolate chips morphed into bowls of cereal and now I can't remember the last time he had a pre-bedtime snack of primarily sugar. (He now realizes that needing food to stay awake is usually a good sign he's tired enough to just go to sleep.)

If you honestly don't have any starches on hand at home, don't let that be what keeps you from starting. Not starting today turns into starting tomorrow, which turns into maybe next month, which as we all know, never happens. Don't let this be you.

Look, in almost every home there is some starch. Use it. Rolled oats? Could be breakfast for dinner! What's that? You don't have a single starch (potatoes, rice, quinoa, pasta) or beans on hand? A quick trip to any grocery store and you could get a bag of rice, a bag of potatoes, and a few cans of beans for under $10. Grab some oats while you're at it and you'll have breakfast and the base for cookies and energy bars covered as well.

No need to buy eggs—one tablespoon of ground flaxseed mixed with three tablespoons of water equal one egg. Simply use this in any baking that calls for eggs. Or, Bob's Red Mill sells an egg replacer. These obviously won't work for making scrambled eggs, but as you'll see later in a recipe, tofu makes a great breakfast scramble that is egg-like.

When we started this journey, my husband was growing a new business, I was working part-time, and four of us were living in a

750-square foot cabin in the woods. Affordability and efficiency were important. As you'll soon see, the time and money you save by eating this way will more than make up for the learning curve in the beginning.

Uh, oh, I forgot about breakfast tomorrow

Okay, you've successfully cleaned out your kitchen and meal prepped for at least one dinner, all with things you already had. Yay you! Before going to bed, think about what your family will eat for breakfast. If it's cereal and you don't already have non-dairy milk on hand, you can have dry cereal, or cereal with orange juice or even water (we've only done this when there is absolutely no other choice, but it works in a pinch). You could also do toast with jam or honey, or a nut butter (or both).

If you have oats, you could make a simple overnight oatmeal.

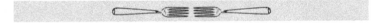

For one serving, start with:

1/2 cup oats
1 cup plant-based milk (could also be water)
1/2 tsp vanilla
Pinch of salt

From there, add whatever else you have and like: 1 Tbsp chia or flaxseeds, 2 Tbsp of nut butter, 1Tbsp unsweetened cocoa powder, 1 teaspoon vanilla, up to 2 Tbsp honey or maple syrup, or raisins/dates/other dried fruit, some shredded coconut, an additional 1/4 cup steel-cut oats for extra chewiness—you get the picture. The sky (or, in this case, the bowl) is the limit.

Make one big batch for the whole family, stir it up, cover it and put it in the fridge for at least four hours and you've got a healthy, filling, tasty breakfast, once again with things you've already got on hand. Or, let everyone have their own containers and add what they'd like to their own oat base. One person may want to add cocoa powder and banana, and another may like cinnamon and raisins.

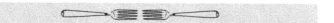

Other lifestyle choices

A word about caffeine and alcohol, for those of you who can't imagine going without that cup of coffee or tea or glass of wine at night—you can rest assured I'm not asking you to give those up. You can find studies arguing both the benefits and harmful effects of coffee and alcohol. While they don't fit under the whole, unprocessed foods category, I'd encourage you to learn more about what they do to your body. I've given up coffee many times and always come back to it because I love it. Recently, I've done the same with alcohol. I would encourage you to think about what these products do for you and why you feel you need them, and then act accordingly.

When I taught the required Nutrition, Self-Esteem, and Exercise class (fondly referred to by the students as 'nutri-sex') at the local university, I was taken aback by the lack of nutritional awareness. When I asked the question, "How many ounces of water do you drink everyday?" I was met with silence. After an awkward pause a student finally said, "I don't drink water. I drink Sunny D in the morning with coffee and Coke in the afternoon."

If it's soda or juice you can't live without, then I'd find a healthier replacement. Soda is filled with sugar (around 10 teaspoons per can)[85] and fruit juices, while having some benefits such as vitamins and nutrients, often times aren't that much better than soda nutritionally speaking, and lack fiber. Instead of orange juice, eat an orange. The fiber in the orange will help your body regulate the natural sugar, absorbing it more slowly.[86]

And what about exercise? Sleep? Healthy relationships? These are all important aspects of a healthy life as well, but not the subject of this book. I will say, it's a myth that you can eat whatever you want as long as you're working out or exercising. Though you may appear healthy on the outside, the "silent killer" (high blood pressure) didn't get that name for no reason.[87] I know two people who lost their dads while they were out for their daily jogs.

I encourage daily exercise—which could be as simple as a 30-minute walk (or three 10-minute walks). The physical and mental benefits are many. Find some type of movement you enjoy, and treat it like a prescription—something you need to do daily. It can be helpful to reframe it as something you *get* to do, rather than something you *have* to do.

---

85   Lindsay Boyers, "How Many Teaspoons of Sugar Are There in a Can of Coke?" Livestrong, updated May 20, 2019, https://www.livestrong.com/article/283136 -how-many-teaspoons-of-sugar-are-there-in-a-can-of-coke/.

86   "Fiber," Harvard School of Public Health, accessed February 27, 2022, https:// www.hsph.harvard.edu/nutritionsource/carbohydrates/fiber/.

87   "Why High Blood Pressure is a 'Silent Killer,'" American Heart Association, updated November 30, 2017, https://www.heart.org/en/health-topics/high-blood-pressure/why-high-blood-pressure-is-a-silent-killer.

It's hard to eat well when you're tired, or stressed. You may need to sleep more, or less (not having caffeine or alcohol could potentially help here as well). You might find less screen time and more interpersonal relationship time helps your overall outlook. All these things are important areas to be explored. Starting to get HAPPY may just give you the motivation you need to make changes in other areas of your life that need some adjusting.

Staying on topic

When you start delving into nutrition, food guidelines, and expert advice, you will find there is a lot of information and research out there and much of it can seem conflicting. I've attempted to give you a solid start to implementing a WFPBNO/HAPPY life—and I've tried to avoid topics that drift off into other areas, mainly because they can act like distractions.

For example, sugar. Which is better: brown sugar, Stevia, maple syrup, date syrup, or molasses? There are arguments supporting them all. But the basic idea would be to eat as many whole, unprocessed foods as possible. So banana (or applesauce or dates) as a sweetener when you bake would be preferable to white sugar (as mentioned above, you're getting more fiber with the whole fruit being used, which is helping your body regulate the absorption of glucose). If your recipe calls for one cup of sugar, use one cup of mashed banana (or applesauce, prune puree, or dates). But using sugar is not off the table. Start by asking yourself whether there is a whole, plant-based food that would work as a replacement.

What about salt? How much is okay? Is none better than some? What if you work out and sweat? Some advocate for no salt intake, but a small amount of salt on foods makes them way more enjoyable, therefore we opt to salt food once it's on our plate—if it's a WFPBNO/HAPPY food. By that I mean at home, I'll salt a sweet potato covered in black beans and kale, but if I'm at a restaurant I don't salt any food because it's, a) processed, and b) highly salted already.

Endless discussion could be had here about transition foods, or the latest vegan version of something. It all comes down to this: is it a whole (as unprocessed as possible) plant-based food? Or is it a highly processed food product, made with lots of other highly processed food products? For example, edamame (soy beans) are a great choice, tofu is a more processed choice, and soy chorizo meat crumbles would be a highly processed choice. Homemade cashew cheese is a great choice, store-bought almond "cream cheese" would be more processed, and vegan cheddar shreds would be highly processed.

Most questions can be answered simply by going back to the question: is it WFPBNO/HAPPY? If the answer is "no," then you can probably find something better for you (and the planet) to consume.

Toss it, throw it, give it, (TTG) but don't hide it

This is your reminder to make a quick decision. Get rid of the food that can cause you harm and start thinking about which meals can work tonight. By cleaning out now, you're helping to ensure your success in this quick 10-day transition.

Tomorrow, we're going to look at taking what your family already loves to eat and making it WFPBNO/HAPPY. Yum!

For fork's sake, LET'S DO THIS!

- Do a TTG session (Toss it, Throw it, Give it away) of your own. As whole food, plant-based, no oil Chef AJ says, "If it's in your house it's in your mouth."[88] After you've cleaned out the fridge and cupboards, take a deep breath and pat yourself on the back.
- If you haven't already, now would be a great time to watch either *Forks Over Knives* or *Gamechangers*.

88   Jolia Sidona Allen, "Chef AJ Shares Her Secrets for Healthy, Plant-Based Weight Loss," Forks Over Knives, July 9, 2018, https://www.forksoverknives.com/how-tos/chef-aj-shares-her-secrets-for-healthy-plant-based-weight-loss/.

DAY 3

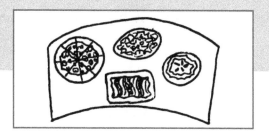

EASY REPLACEMENTS

*"Knowledge is knowing that a tomato is a fruit;
wisdom is not putting it in a fruit salad."*
—Miles Kington[89]

So, you've done the great clean out, now what are you going to eat that everybody will love? Your family already loves certain foods. They might even ask for them on their birthday and now it's possible that they can't have them. Thoughts cross your mind as to when you will experience your first family mutiny. The truth is, there's no reason you can't achieve those same flavors in new ways, and some new and different flavors will almost certainly become new favorites.

It's helpful to start with a list. Ask your family what they like to eat and think back to what you end up eating most often.

---

89   Mark Minkler, "The Tomato Philosophy," November 16, 2017, https://limmereducation.com/article/the-tomato-philosophy/.

It's helpful to have buy-in from everyone, and it's helpful to make HAPPY versions of everyone's favorites, especially in the beginning.

Let it be a surprise at first, but don't yell, "Surprise!"

"I can't believe you liked those enchiladas, the main ingredient was sweet potatoes!"

"Wow, that chocolate smoothie had a cup of frozen peas in it and you didn't even taste them!"

It happened often that I'd make a really tasty smoothie, or try a new enchilada recipe or dessert and my somewhat picky eater son would really love it. I was so excited he liked it I'd blurt out something like the phrases above. Suddenly, the love for that new recipe would fly out the window. Just knowing what it was made of ruined it.

That's an inside joke for my son, who's now 18. He'll comment that he really liked something and I'll ask him, "Do you want to know what was in it?" Nine times out of 10 he wants to know now. But in the beginning, I had to let go of my desire to point out that he was joyfully eating some food he claimed to hate.

Where do I even start?

Start with dinner, since dinner usually takes the most effort. Ask everyone what their favorite meal is. On our family favorites dinner list were:

- Macaroni and cheese
- Lasagna

- Enchiladas
- Pasta
- Mashed potatoes and gravy
- Meat loaf
- Burritos
- Quesadillas
- Chili and cornbread
- Burgers
- Nachos

Finding WFPBNO/HAPPY recipes for these family favorites wasn't hard. We made them a few times, tweaking them and finding our favorite version, and now they're often on meal rotation.

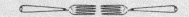

Macaroni and not cheese

If it's macaroni with cheese that your kids love (ours sure did), then give this a try. And it's not just for kids, adults love it too! This is our go-to "cheese" sauce—there are gazillions online, including nut-free versions.

I most often use The Full Helping's **Go-to Cashew Cheese** recipe (thefullhelping.com).

1 cup raw cashews (soaked two hours to overnight if you are going to use a blender, or pour boiling water over them and let them sit for 10 minutes if you forgot to soak them)
2 Tbsp nutritional yeast, sometimes called "nooch"
2 Tbsp lemon juice
¼-¾ tsp garlic powder

½ tsp salt

¼ tsp black pepper

¼–½ cup water as needed.[90]

Simply put all the ingredients into a blender and blend until you get a smooth consistency. Pour over cooked pasta and—boom—you're done. I often toss in frozen peas, or broccoli—use any vegetable your family likes. Toss in a few more vegetables, top with bread crumbs, herbs, salt, and pepper and bake at 425 degrees for 20 to 25 minutes and you've got a yummy, comforting casserole for dinner.

"But raw cashews are expensive!" I can hear you saying from here. We'll get to shopping soon, but I promise you, when you remove all the dairy, meat, oil, and processed foods you were purchasing, you can buy a lot of raw cashews and still come out ahead. More than once, I've been slightly terrified at the size of the pile in my grocery cart when approaching check out only to be pleasantly reminded that starches, beans, and fresh and frozen produce cost way less by volume than meat, dairy, oil, and processed foods.

Pasta is an easy dinner, with either red sauce and veggies, or a cashew cheese and veggies. There are even fettucine alfredo recipes that use potato to make a HAPPY creamy sauce. My daughter used to make it quite often; it's great for a cold day or anytime you're craving something creamy.

90 "Go-to Cashew Cheese Recipe," The Full Helping, updated September 16, 2021, https://www.thefullhelping.com/go-to-cashew-cheese-recipe/.

Pick one or two of your family's favorite recipes, and see if you can make it HAPPY. It might be easiest to just Google "vegan lasagna recipe" or "whole food plant-based chicken pot pie recipe" to see if there are already recipes out there that you could use. If not, start by swapping the meat out for some other plant protein (such as beans, lentils, or tofu). Try omitting the oil. Use plant-based milks instead of cream. Replace cheese with HAPPY cheese.

Macaroni and cheese was a treat at our house. Since it was no longer coming out of a box on rare occasions, I let my kids pick which shape of pasta they would like in their macaroni and cheese. Little kids usually enjoy having a say in what they eat, so this proved to be a hit. Sometimes they'd pick shell-shaped pasta, or sometimes bow-tie. They loved having frozen peas added as well, and we even experimented with other vegetables of their choice.

Tacos and tostadas were a great meal to make HAPPY as well, for much the same reason I think—the kids got to pick what they wanted to put in them or on them. Instead of shredded cheese, sour cream, and ground beef with seasoning, I'd make some HAPPY cheese, slice up an avocado, and either season beans with some cumin and chili powder, or sauté (in water or broth) onions and then crumble in tofu and add taco seasoning. Chopped red and/or green pepper, onion, cilantro, tomato, some shredded cabbage or lettuce and—voila!—a dinner everyone loves.

After eating healthy and plant-powered meals at home, the old versions of these favorites didn't taste as good. The kids would be excited to eat mac-n-cheese or some snack food at a friend's house, only to return to say it didn't taste as good as they remembered.

Comfort food with extra added comfort

There are some foods that just sound like home and immediately feel comforting. In a conversation with my daughter recently, I told her that tomato soup paired with grilled cheese, and tuna melts were some foods I occasionally missed. I asked her what food she missed (we started eating this way when she was eight). Her answer surprised me. She thought for a minute, and then said she didn't have any non-HAPPY meals she missed. The comforting meals she associated with home and often craved were all plant-based meals.

For every comforting meal you love, I assure you there's a HAPPY version you will either love or come to love soon. Lasagna was a family favorite. After a few tries we found a plant-based version that we ended up liking even more than the SAD version we used to eat. Chef AJ, a plant-based chef, culinary instructor, speaker, and author who has been eating plants exclusively for over 43 years,[91] has an amazing plant-based lasagna recipe, which is our favorite.[92] See www.forforkssakebook.com for the link.

Mashed potatoes and gravy are easy to make WFPBNO/ HAPPY. Make mashed potatoes as you normally would, but instead of adding milk, butter, or cream, simply add a plant-based milk or some of the drained potato water. Check out my website for our favorite gravy recipe. It's delicious and can serve as an entire meal over mashed potatoes or rice, or even pasta.

And what about desserts? This book isn't filled with recipes, but if you are not too overwhelmed to start digging through the

---

91   "Meet Chef AJ," Chef AJ, accessed February 25, 2022, https://www.chefaj.com/about.

92   Chef AJ, "Chef AJ's Disappearing Lasagna," PB Life, April 19, 2015, https://pblife. org/recipes/chef-ajs-disappearing-lasagna/.

internet for recipes on Day 3, go to my website www.forforks-sakebook.com and you'll find myriads of meals to try that may replace those you love. You'll be amazed when you start looking at the wide variety of options out there. The most difficult part will be deciding what you want to try first.

Overwhelmed by self-replacements?

Here's a comforting thought when you're starting out and attempting to create entirely new meals: the HAPPY lifestyle is offered at many restaurants that cater to this niche. When you see their menus and what they have created to replace your old favorites and expose you to whole new tastes, you'll feel like you're part of a larger community.

Search online in your locality for "vegan, plant-based" and a wide array of new restaurants will be available. You may not find anything listed under HAPPY restaurants, but deep down you know that's what they're thinking. Don't worry, we'll delve into eating out later—you'll have plenty of options.

Help, I'm running errands and starving! Where can I eat?

It happens to all of us at some point—we end up far from home without WFPBNO/HAPPY food on hand and we need something fast. What to do?

If you're near a grocery store with a deli, have them make a veggie sandwich on sourdough bread (or whole-wheat without oil). Use hummus or avocado instead of mayonnaise, then add all the veggies you like. Same goes for Subway—you can load up on all the veggies and add some mustard and you've got a great meal.

At Wendy's, you could get a baked potato (just hold the dairy and meat toppings). You'll likely be surprised at how satisfying a plain baked potato can be. Stuck at a burger joint? No patty, but all the veggies on a bun works in a pinch.

Years ago, we drove seven hours to visit my parents and stopped for gas near an In-N-Out Burger. I ordered a "veggie burger," which was the bun, sauce, and veggies (since they don't have a veggie patty). They must get this request often, because they didn't bat an eye. It was surprisingly tasty, and I didn't miss the meat or cheese. This was our first road trip splurge in some time, and a far cry from our first trip to In-N-Out in 2006 when we excitedly ordered cheeseburgers, fries, and milkshakes.

Early in our transition to plant-based eating, when we'd eat out my husband would order a bacon burger with all the fixin's and sub out a veggie patty for the burger but keep the bacon. He just couldn't give up the bacon. This seriously confused a few wait staffers, but when he explained he was trying but just couldn't give up the bacon yet, they 100% understood.

I often order fish tacos, but instead of fish I ask for avocado. So I get the corn tortillas, shredded cabbage, pico de gallo, and avocado and (usually) sauce, which makes an amazing treat for a meal out. Beans in a burrito with veggies—you can make almost anything work. You'll be getting a little added oil most likely, but you don't have to throw in the HAPPY towel.

Ultimately, you'll probably remember to keep some easy to-go food on hand in the future. I try to take some fresh fruit or veggies with me when I leave the house in case I get hungry when I'm out and about. A homemade sandwich, pumpkin seeds, HAPPY muffins, or cookies have also saved me when I was away from home. As one woman who has successfully eaten this way for years said recently, "I'm always pimping it when I leave the house. You know, 'Potato In My Purse.'"

What about lunches?

Lunches take moderate effort. People vary as to whether they prefer variety or they enjoy the same lunch (peanut butter and jelly anyone?) every day. Sandwiches and wraps (like chickpea instead of tuna, or hummus and veggies) work well here, as do leftovers from dinner, and soups and salads.

Kids' lunches can be super easy (see above). And when some teacher or parent asks where they get their protein, you can rest easy knowing they're getting plenty of protein eating WFPBNO/HAPPY.

A sandwich or wrap or burrito with some veggie sticks and hummus, or leftover mac-n-cashew cheese, or leftover soup, some fresh fruit or a 100% fruit strip bar, no oil crackers, all work well. I often made a WFPBNO/HAPPY cookie or dessert to add in, and the kids would ask for extra since their friends enjoyed them as well.

A longtime favorite lunch goodie was "peanut butter balls" (though any nut butter would work).

Happy Peanut Butter Balls

½-1 cup peanut butter with enough honey added to stir both easily (about ¼–½ cup)

1/4–1/2 cup oats—or 1 Tbsp ground flaxseeds with 1 Tbsp–1/4 cup sesame seeds—or all three
1 tsp vanilla
Pinch of salt

Mix all the ingredients in small bowl and roll into little balls. If you'd like, roll in shredded coconut or stick a chocolate chip on top. Place in freezer for a few hours. You can pull them out to put in lunches, or have as a snack. (They're also amazing with a cup of coffee.)

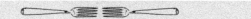

What about protein?

Plant-based dietitian and author Julieanna Hever recently posted on social media (10/1/21):

"5 Facts About Protein:
- We don't need protein. We need a few essential amino acids
- All plants contain all amino acids in different ratios
- Protein is not a food group
- Protein is not meat"[93]

There were a few facts that changed everything for me when learning about whole food plant-based eating. The role of animal protein in feeding cancer was one of them. (The fact that I don't have to get pancreatic cancer like my uncle and grandfather even though I have the same (APOe) genes was comforting to say the least.)

---

93   plantdietitian, Twitter post, September 25, 2021, https://mobile.twitter.com/plantdietitian/status/1441792183963553808.

Starting to learn these things also made me mad. Why don't more people know this? Why is dairy subsidized by our government? Why are manufacturers of food products made with animal proteins allowed to put pink lids on their products and sponsor breast cancer awareness when what they sell actually feeds cancer tumors? We need only five to 14 percent of our calories to come from protein. The average U.S. intake of protein is at 15 to 25 percent.

Excess protein hurts our bones, kidneys, and liver. Getting just 10 percent of calories from protein has been found to be enough for endurance athletes.[94] You can get all the protein you need from plants (beans, grains, nuts, seeds). Broccoli contains more protein per calorie than steak, and spinach per calorie is about equal to chicken and fish. Asparagus, artichokes, potatoes, sweet potatoes and brussels sprouts all contain about 4 to 5 grams of protein per cooked cup.[95]

Dr. T. Colin Campbell's research has shown that casein (animal protein) fed at higher than recommended intakes promotes cancer. At 10 percent, there was a sharp increase in foci cell clusters (early tumor developments). However, soy and wheat plant proteins even at 20 percent did not cause tumor growth. Did you catch that? Twice as much plant protein had no adverse effect on tumor development.

The rumor that soy is bad for you and raises estrogen levels to a dangerous level, especially in boys? That's a myth. Soy is

---

94   Michaela Karlsen, "How Much Protein Do We Need? RDA vs. Dietary Guidelines," updated January 7, 2019, https://nutritionstudies.org/how-much -protein-do-we-need-rda-vs-dietary-guidelines/.

95   "The 18 Best Protein Sources for Vegans and Vegetarians," Healthline, accessed February 27, 2022, https://www.healthline.com/nutrition/protein-for-vegans -vegetarians#TOC_TITLE_HDR_3.

beneficial and even more protective in kids[96, 97, 98]—so go ahead and eat the soybeans, soy milk, tofu, and tempeh. Jackie Busse, MD, a pediatrician in Santa Cruz, California says the more plants kids eat, the less asthma they have. Children raised plant-based have reduced risk for heart disease, cancer, obesity, diabetes, and other conditions.

What about protein powders? These are powdered forms of protein—typically milk or eggs, as well as plant sources like soy, peas, hemp, or rice. The first problem with these are that we don't need them. If you're eating enough calories through a variety of whole plant-based foods, then you're eating enough protein. The second problem with protein powder is that they are ultra-processed. The protein is isolated from the rest of the food's components (carbohydrates and fats) through chemical processing and then often mixed with other ingredients (flavor-masking agents, for example).[99] This processing takes out all the "good stuff," such as fiber, vitamins, minerals, antioxidants, and essential fatty acids, which our body needs and uses, and introduces potential contamination with toxins like heavy metals.[100]

You can rest easy knowing that as long as you're eating whole, plant-based foods, you're getting enough protein.

96   Melissa Halas, "Is Soy Safe for Kids?" SuperKids Nutrition, accessed March 25, 2022, https://www.superkidsnutrition.com/is-soy-safe-for-kids/.

97   Mark Messina et al., "Health Impact of Childhood and Adolescent Soy Consumption." Nutrition Reviews 75, no. 7. (2017): 500-515.

98   "Is Soy Healthy for Kids?" Plant Based Juniors, March 23, 2020. https://plantbasedjuniors.com/soy-healthy-for-kids/.

99   Theresa "Sam" Houghton, "Protein Isolates: Do They Have a Place in a Whole Food, Plant-Based Diet?" T. Colin Campbell Center for Nutrition Studies, October 27, 2021, https://nutritionstudies.org/protein-isolates-do-they-have-a-place-in-a-whole-food-plant-based-diet/.

100   "The Hidden Dangers of Protein Powders." Harvard Health Publishing, April 10, 2020. https://www.health.harvard.edu/staying-healthy/the-hidden-dangers-of-protein-powders.

The most important meal of the day: breakfast

One of our favorite breakfasts when we had chickens was a fried egg on toast with slices of avocado. It took a while to stop missing the egg. But, we started trying different kinds of avocado toast—adding not just salt and pepper, but some radishes or pickled onions, or both. Next came the addition of sriracha sauce or hummus or baba ganoush or sliced tomato, cucumber, and arugula. You're going to start identifying foods you love that, with just a few changes, you can still enjoy.

A note here: we live in California where avocados are in almost every store year-round and are decently affordable. My husband and I both grew up in Washington state where avocados were expensive. We would have guacamole every once in a while, but neither of us ever remember adding avocado to anything.

When we lived in Hawaii, we had a papaya tree in the yard of the house we rented, so we enjoyed a lot of tropical fruit that we otherwise wouldn't have bought. Though we'd never been big fans of brussels sprouts, here in California we learned from locals how to cook them and they are one of our favorite foods now.

All that is to say, explore and enjoy what is available to you locally. Though we no longer eat meat, if my brother catches and smokes salmon, I enjoy it. Remember, it's what you do 90 percent of the time that is going to make the biggest difference in the long run.

For breakfasts during the week, we keep it simple. Oatmeal with toppings such as chopped apples, bananas, raisins, or cranberries, frozen or fresh berries, and nuts. Sometimes nut butter is a go to, or savory (avocado/hummus/veggies) or sweet (nut butter with jam) toast.

On the weekends with more time, we'll make tofu scrambles, pancakes, waffles or scones. Check out www.forforkssakebook. com for a HAPPY tofu scramble recipe, as well as easy pancake and waffle recipes.

Prepping to be HAPPY

On weekends (or anytime you tend to have a few hours), batch cooking really helps make weekday life easier. If you cook up a pot of beans and a pot of rice, you now have the base for at least three dinners. You could make enchiladas, burritos, bowls, and soup, all from those two main ingredients you precooked and have ready to use.

While the rice and beans are cooking, you can chop up onions and peppers so they're ready to use in recipes. Slice or cut bell peppers, carrots, celery, and radishes to dip in hummus for snacks or to put in sandwiches or wraps or on top of bowls. Or you could roast a bunch of root vegetables (some combination of potatoes, sweet potatoes, turnips, beets, parsnips, garlic, onion, broccoli and cauliflower). Now you have a side, or a bowl topper, or a wrap filling. You could pre-make a double batch of cashew cheese sauce to drizzle on the enchiladas, put on pasta or pizza or pour over the roasted vegetables.

This hour or two of prepping healthy, HAPPY foods will keep you from being in the danger zone. You know, that place when you get home and are starving and there's nothing good to eat and your resolve is low and so you'll eat anything or order out? Do yourself and your family a favor and get ahead on prepping a few simple things and you'll be thanking yourself later in the week.

Let's get the groceries... But how? But where?

Now that you have a list of favorite meals, it's time to head to the grocery store (or to your favorite grocery store online). As an adult, you've likely shopped at a grocery store thousands of times, but there are a few tricks that will make shopping WFPBNO a little easier. We'll get to that next.

For fork's sake, LET'S DO THIS!

- Make a list of favorite meals you want to try.
- Make a grocery list of what you need to make said meals.
- Head to the store!

DAY 4

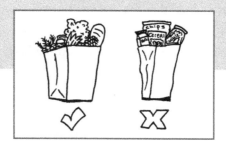

QUICK SHOPPING GUIDE: HOW TO BUY MORE AND SAVE MONEY

"**GIVE A MAN** a fish and you feed him for a day; teach a man to fish and he'll empty the seas by 2050 and we'll all die. You should teach a man to cook lentils."[101]

This is the moment of truth. You have an idea of what to buy, but where will you find this stuff? You may be wondering, "What if my grocery store doesn't have any of it?"

Keeping it simple

I'd finished teaching a yoga class and stopped at the grocery store to grab a veggie panini before picking up my kids from

---

101 @ancientleolester, Twitter post, December 25, 2018, "https://twitter.com/ ancienleolester/status/1077494569955221504.

preschool. The high schooler in front of me held a brown box from the salad bar. The checker weighed it and said, "That will be 19 dollars and 12 cents." The color drained from the young man's face as he mumbled he didn't have that much money. She kindly explained that the mashed potatoes were priced by the pound at the salad bar, hence the price. She told him he didn't have to purchase them, and he left, embarrassed and by the looks of it, without lunch. It made me think, how did we learn how to shop?

You've cleaned out your kitchen, and you've got a list of your family's favorite recipes. You've got your wallet and hopefully your reusable bags and it's time to go shopping—what do you buy? And where do you go?

First off, as long as you're not buying "junk" vegan replacements (by which I mean prepackaged products that took a machine to make) you're going to save a lot of money.

Although vegan deli meats, vegan cheeses, vegan ice cream and let's not forget Oreos ("but they're vegan!" my kids used to point out) may not contain animal products, they are highly processed. More on this in a minute. We're aiming to buy whole plant-based foods.

By taking out the meat, fish, oil, cheese, milk, yogurt, cottage cheese, and ice cream, you've likely eliminated the most expensive grocery items. Fresh fruits and vegetables, grains and legumes, and even nuts will be less expensive than all the animal products you used to buy. You don't need a Whole Foods or a specialty market to eat this way. Any conventional supermarket or grocery store will have what we're looking for. There are people who eat this way buying what they need from dollar stores, so don't let your perceived lack of access to food dissuade you from giving this a go.

"Transition" foods and their place

If you tend to be more black and white, sticking to your entirely WFPBNO/HAPPY diet, then so-called "transition foods" may not be enticing. However, for some people, they help ease the journey into a new way of eating, bridging the gap between eating meat-lovers' pizza and baked tofu sandwiches. The transition foods I'm speaking of are highly processed vegan substitutes for foods you are used to eating. So, Beyond Burgers or Impossible Burgers instead of a meat burger. Soy ice cream instead of dairy ice cream. Almond cheese slices instead of cheese made from dairy.

Though better in terms of having less casein and saturated fat, these products aren't usually a whole lot better for you than their counterparts. Often they contain oil, sometimes large amounts of it. They usually consist of broken down and rearranged food parts, such as soy protein isolate. Better to eat actual edamame (soy beans), or baked tofu (which is less processed) than a product that contains highly processed soy.

That being said, some people find it convenient and don't mind the cost of using replacement foods to help them start to make the change. Very honestly, I get it, but in this 10-day book I'm trying to move you quickly to HAPPY and I don't want you to slip back to SAD. Do your best to avoid processed vegan foods.

If you are going to eat transition foods, just make sure you eventually make the change if health benefits are what you're going for. There are plenty of unhealthy vegans, even though they're not eating animal products. They are instead eating heavily processed foods rich in oils, salt, sugar, and substances derived originally from actual food.

Julieanna Hever, a registered dietitian and author who has been in the plant-based world for decades, recently told Rip Esselstyn on his Plantstrong podcast that she is now seeing vegan clients with the same medical issues she used to see in people who ate SAD.[102] Because they are consuming so many processed vegan foods, many are having issues with high blood pressure, heart disease, and diabetes. So, aim for whole plant-based no oil foods to be the basis of what you eat.

If you're making the change from the SAD to WFPBNO/HAPPY for health reasons, treat transition foods like other high fat foods (coconut, avocado, tofu, nuts) and use them occasionally, rather than daily. Or have them only on special occasions. For example, my kids love non-dairy ice creams, so we sometimes have them on family birthdays.

There are also WFPBNO/HAPPY versions that can help if you're missing certain foods. Carrot dogs initially sounded ridiculous to me, but I have to say we've been impressed after making them a few times.

Yonanas Ice Cream can be a tasty substitute for ice cream lovers. (This is a home ice cream maker that produces a frozen yogurt type ice cream using just frozen bananas and whatever else you

---

102 Rip Esselstyn and Julieanna Hever, "120: Rip Esselstyn Talks Food and Family
     with Julieanna Hever on the 'Choose You Now' Podcast," November 25, 2021, in
     Plantstrong Podcast, podcast, MP3 Audio, 28:22, https://www.plantstrongpodcast.
     com/blog/choose-you-now-replay.

add.) And our all-time favorite substitute—cashew cheese. In the last year we probably have eaten cashew cheese at least once a month. So, while hot dogs, ice cream, and cheese may be out, WFPBNO/HAPPY versions of them may help you get through a season of missing them.

I'm assuming you already have all the staples you need (flour, sugar, baking powder, salt). Things to start adding to your cart if you don't already have them could be:

- Oatmeal (rolled oats)
- Ground flax seed (to use as an egg replacer)
- Grains such as brown rice
- Quinoa
- Polenta
- Whole wheat pastas

In addition to fresh or frozen vegetables and fruits, you may want to add some nuts and seeds. If you're buying nut butters (peanut, almond, cashew, sunflower, etc.) make sure they don't have added oils. Same goes for salad dressings. There are a few that don't have added oils, but make sure to read the label. You can always make your own dressing as well.

Like tahini? Equal parts tahini and lemon juice, with water added to a consistency you like, plus some garlic powder a little dill and some salt and pepper and you've got a tasty dressing.

Hummus watered down with a little lemon juice and/or mustard and herbs of your liking works well too. You get the idea—experiment a little and find an easy dressing that you like. Can't give up the ranch habit? There are some great WFPBNO ranch recipes on the internet, as well as Caesar salad dressing recipes.

You don't have to buy everything in bulk and cook it yourself. Especially in the beginning, if it's helpful, buy pre-cooked canned beans, or frozen vegetables. Polenta, which is like cornmeal, comes in a tube, ready to use, and makes a great base for a meal. Just be sure to read labels no matter what you buy. You may find that those no-fat, vegetarian refried beans have added oil.

Non-food shopping tips to stay HAPPY

Eat BEFORE you go shopping, especially now. It will help you avoid impulse buys that sound really good when you're hungry.

The biggest key is staying to the perimeter, or outer edges of the grocery store. Wandering aisles won't help you here. Most especially, avoid snack food sections (particularly if your kids are with you!). Have a list and stick to it, unless of course some produce or something you use often is on sale or special. And don't forget your reusable bags!

What to look for when buying produce

> *"An average serving of vegetables may cost roughly four times more than the average serving of junk food, but those veggies have been calculated to average twenty-four times more nutrition."*
> — Dr. Michael Greger, How Not to Die[103]

After helping me move into my first house with roommates where I'd be cooking for myself my junior year of college, my mom and I went to the store. I'd helped shop all the time while

---

103   Michael Greger, *How Not to Die: Discover the Foods Scientifically Proven to Prevent and Reverse Disease* (New York: Flatiron Books, 2015).

growing up and had learned to smell cantaloupe for ripeness like my grandmother did and I picked firm potatoes with no sprouting "eyes." But I realized the moment I went to grab some broccoli that I didn't know how to pick it—what specifically was I looking for in good broccoli? Firm, not soft crowns, my mother told me.

Fresh, colorful produce is full of antioxidants, vitamins, and minerals. You can ask people in the produce department how to pick the best produce. You can also ask them how certain produce is usually prepared. Or if you don't want to ask a person, you can always ask the internet. What do you look for when choosing fresh asparagus? Not sure how to prepare beet greens? Just ask the internet or come to my website and look for the link on veggie buying tips.

For a few years, we split a CSA (community supported agriculture) box with another family. With small kids, we didn't think we'd be able to eat all the veggies and fruit that came each week. Every other week I'd drive with the kids to the house that had all the boxes of produce piled up. We'd grab our box, and sometimes there was a "grab box" that had extra bunches of produce where you could take one, or exchange something you didn't want, or leave some type of produce you didn't think you'd use. We'd read the list and look in our box to see what we were getting that week and make any exchanges.

Sometimes there'd be a vegetable in the box that we'd never heard of. Have you seen Romanesco broccoli? These days it's available at grocery stores, but over 10 years ago when we had some in our CSA box, we laughed upon seeing it and wondered what prehistoric plant it was. We were introduced to tomatillos, and persimmons, and probably six different types of peppers. Thankfully, the list that came with the box had recipe suggestions, which was helpful in identifying what to do with unknown fruits and vegetables. The CSA box was a good way to get healthy, organic produce while supporting a nearby farm.

Then our community started a farmers market. We committed to going every week for a year (it was year-round for one year). We wanted to support the market and see what local produce was available throughout the seasons. (We learned that brussels sprouts, butternut squash, and lemons seemed to be the local winter staples around here.)

A few years in, we started riding our bikes as a family to the farmers market. Besides all the fresh fruits and vegetables grown nearby, there was live music and a bakery that had oil-free bread. By this time, our kids had favorites they wanted from the farmers market each week depending on the season. From strawberries that tasted like sunshine to the brussels sprouts we'd all come to love, the kids would now ask for fresh produce. New favorites were Nantes carrots, green peppers, tomatoes, nectarines, and peaches.

Frozen fruits and veggies are just great

I like to use fresh veggies as much as possible, but a number of times I've had people tell me that their fruits and veggies would go bad too fast. Especially as they were getting used to the new way of eating.

Frozen fruits and veggies are harvested at the peak of freshness and are usually blanched to help preserve all their nutrients, so no need to worry about them being substandard. Shopping for frozen items may take you into the center of the grocery store, so stay focused on those fruits and veggies and turn a blind eye to all those processed packaged meals nearby.

Don't panic—you don't have to buy all organic

As we've established, it's not just your body that benefits from these changes, it's also your wallet. With the money you are saving by cutting out meat, fish, dairy, and oil, you can afford to buy all kinds of vegetables and fruits, grains and beans. Even organic produce.

Consumer Reports found in 2015 that, on average, organic foods were 47 percent more expensive. However, depending on where you shop and what for, some items such as organic lettuce, carrots and maple syrup were the same price or less than their conventional counterparts. Let's suppose for 2,000 calories per day it costs around $2.50 more for organic than for conventional food.[104] That's still less than a drink from Starbucks or a bag of chips. I understand that not everyone is buying a Starbucks drink (or a bag of chips) every day, but it's worth considering what you're willing to spend money on. If you can't afford organic at all, don't stress. I'll give you some pointers below as to when and if organic makes sense for different foods.

Eating organic helps to limit the amount of pesticides and chemicals on your food. Fewer chemicals means reducing your risk of cancer and other diseases, but you don't have to buy all organic. In fact, if you can't buy organic at all, don't panic!

Dr. Greger states on nutritionfacts.org that, "there is a clear consensus in the scientific community that the health benefits

---

104 "The Cost of Organic Food," ConsumerReports.org, March 19, 2015, https://www.consumerreports.org/cro/news/2015/03/cost-of-organic-food/index.htm.

from consuming fruits and vegetables outweigh any potential risks from pesticide residues."[105] In other words, it's better to eat non-organic fruits and vegetables than to skip those vegetables just because they aren't organic. Simply be sure to rinse your produce with water before using it.

It's not always worth it to buy organic. Some foods, such as those on the Clean 15 list, when tested, aren't that different from their organic counterparts. Depending on the year's crops, perennial fruits and vegetables on the Clean 15 list include:

- Avocado
- Sweet corn
- Pineapple
- Onion
- Papaya
- Sweet peas (frozen)
- Eggplant
- Asparagus
- Broccoli
- Cabbage
- Kiwi
- Cauliflower
- Mushrooms
- Honeydew melon
- Cantaloupe[106]

105 Michael Greger, "The Best Way to Wash Fruit and Vegetables," NutritionFacts.org, April 20, 2017, https://nutritionfacts.org/2017/04/20/the-best-way-to-wash-fruit-and-vegetables/.

106 Elizabeth Rider, "Updated Dirty Dozen and Clean 15 (2021)," Elizabeth Rider, accessed February 26, 2022, https://www.elizabethrider.com/dirty-dozen-clean-15/.

In contrast, the Dirty Dozen are foods that are worth buying organic if you can. These produce, when put to the same wash test still have pesticide residue on them. The Dirty Dozen usually lead with:

- Strawberries
- Spinach
- Kale, collard and mustard greens
- Nectarines
- Apples
- Grapes
- Cherries
- Peaches
- Pears
- Bell and hot peppers
- Tomatoes
- Celery[107]

We're attempting to eat whole plant-based food that is free of chemicals. But it bears repeating that eating a piece of washed fruit or vegetable that is not organic will still be better for you than not eating it just because it isn't organic. That conventionally grown apple in your hand will still be better for you than a snack bag of chips.

On the planetary side of things, voting with your dollars by buying organic helps retailers know that you want products with fewer chemicals and pesticides in them. More people demanding organic produce helps drive down the costs associated with becoming organic. Keeping chemicals out of our food and water is no joke. The runoff from agricultural chemicals and factory farms

---

107 Ibid.

is decimating coastal areas, creating dead zones where everything from fish and crab to coral are dying.[108, 109, 110]

As mentioned before, other options for obtaining fresh produce are CSAs and local farmers markets.

Or, as a fun activity, grow something yourself. This doesn't have to be a quarter acre farm. You could build or buy a farm box, or stick a tomato plant or some herbs in your yard or in a small pot on your window sill. Kids, especially, love seeing how things grow and like to help water and then eat what they've grown. Additionally, there is some amazing brain science behind growing a tomato to completion (feel-good chemicals in the brain fire off as your reward for all that watering and waiting).

A note from experience: if you plant mint, put it in a pot. One year we planted mint in a side garden. Within a couple of years it had spread to cover every possible inch of soil surrounding it, coming up 20 feet from where it was originally planted. We discovered some fun recipes to try and use all that mint, but it took a few years to get rid of it.

You have just taken a huge, committed step

Look at you, dear reader! You're making healthy choices for yourself and your family! Good on you! Next, while hoping to

108   Scott Thill, "Largest-Ever Gulf Dead Zone Reveals Stark Impacts of Industrial Agriculture," Civil Eats, accessed February 25, 2022, https://civileats.com/2017/08/03/largest-ever-gulf-dead-zone-reveals-stark-impacts-of-industrial-agriculture/amp/.

109   Oliver Milman, "Meat Industry Blamed for Largest-ever 'Dead Zone' in Gulf of Mexico," The Guardian, August 1, 2017,https://amp.theguardian.com/environment/2017/aug/01/meat-industry-dead-zone-gulf-of-mexico-environment-pollution.

110   Ian Angus, "Dead Zones: Industrial Agriculture versus Ocean Life," Resilience, August 14, 2020, https://www.resilience.org/stories/2020-08-14/dead-zones-industrial-agriculture-versus-ocean-life/

bypass glazed eyes, we'll explore ways of responding when people inevitably ask why you're making the change from the SAD to HAPPY.

For fork's sake, LET'S DO THIS!

- Go to the grocery store (or online) and get what you need. While you're at it, add some new fruits or veggies to snack on.
- You went shopping, way to go, you! Did you find everything you needed? Is there another store or somewhere online or a farmers market or CSA you'd like to try? Find out when they're open, and make it an outing. Or can you find a WFPBNO/HAPPY buddy who'd like to go in on a big bag of dried beans or rice, or a CSA box?

DAY 5

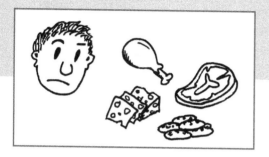

WHY IT'S SO HARD TO NOT EAT THE SAD (COMMON PITFALLS)

"It's not that some people have willpower and some people don't. It's that some people are ready to change and others are not."
—James Gordon, MD[111]

AFTER FINDING OUT my son had high cholesterol at age 10—even though we'd been eating vegan (but not HAPPY) for a few years—we talked with our doctor and decided to do a "no added fat for nine weeks" trial to see if we could lower his cholesterol by cutting out peanut butter and avocado (and any other fat) rather than putting him on medication.

---

111 Verne Varona, *Nature's Cancer-Fighting Foods: Prevent and Reverse the Most Common Forms of Cancer Using the Proven Power of Whole Food and Self-Healing Strategies* (New York: Penguin, 2001), 10.

We packed uber healthy lunches for school, and at least twice a week when I went to pick him up from school, he'd be carrying a brownie, or cookie, or some other "treat" his class had been given. These were from a birthday that was celebrated, or from the teacher as a reward for being nice when they'd had a sub. I knew that treats and parties happened at school, I just didn't realize how often. Being the sweet kid he is, my son would have a forlorn look on his face as he handed the treat to his sister, having saved it all day to give it to her. (Side note: my kids have way more discipline than I do.)

About 10 days into the nine-week cholesterol lowering experiment, we had whole wheat pitas for dinner with hummus and fresh chopped veggies in them (something we'd had many times before). My son took a bite and exclaimed, "These red peppers are SO sweet! They are SO good!"

He thought I'd made the pitas differently somehow that time, and kept saying how amazing they were. It took me a few minutes to realize what had happened, but then I explained to him that his taste buds had changed. That sweet, red pepper tasted sweet because it was, and because he hadn't had excessively sweetened cookies or brownies, his taste buds were recognizing natural sweetness again.

His cholesterol at the end of the nine weeks? Perfect. He unintentionally lost 10% of his body weight as well, eating whole, HAPPY foods until he was full.

It's not just the food, it's also you

Another thing that makes transitioning from a SAD to a HAPPY diet hard is the acquired tastes we all have from eating the SAD for years. Our taste buds love sugar and salt and fat. In fact, that combination of sugar, salt, and fat sets off fireworks of chemicals in our brains. Dr. Douglas J. Lisle, author of *The Pleasure Trap* says, "By causing artificially intensive releases of dopamine within the brain's pleasure centers, these substances create a deceptively intense, short-term feeling of well-being."[112] For biological reasons, seeking calorie-dense foods has helped us survive as a species. At first, it's quite the shock to not be getting those acquired tastes filled with each meal. However, the good news is, our tastes change, and they change rapidly.

Our tastebuds quite literally change about every two weeks.[113] The average person has around 10,000 taste buds, but as you get older they don't all get replaced. An older person may have only 5,000 working taste buds, so certain foods don't taste as strong.[114] This explains why your grandmother can drink a smokey Scotch and not bat an eye, and why a three-year-old may not initially love sauerkraut. This also means that, like my son, about two weeks into changing your diet you will start to notice how sweet your apples or grapes or a raw red pepper taste. Once you allow your tastes to recalibrate to natural sweetness and saltiness (with salt added only to things you cook from scratch at home) you'll be amazed at how flavorful real whole plant-based HAPPY food tastes.

Transitioning to WFPBNO/HAPPY is not meant to be a suffer-fest. One of the greatest things about eating this way for me was learning to eat to satiety, or to fullness. Once, when my

112 Douglas J. Lisle and Alan Goldhamer, *The Pleasure Trap: Mastering the Hidden Force that Undermines Health and Happiness* (Marshfield, MA: Healthy Living Publications, 2003), 158.

113 Elizabeth Bacharach, "How Often Do Your Taste Buds Change?" *Women's Health*, January 17, 2019, https://www.womenshealthmag.com/food/a25838847/how-often-do-your-taste-buds-change/.

114 Natalie Jacewicz, "Why Taste Buds Dull As We Age," The Salt, May 5, 2017, https://www.npr.org/sections/thesalt/2017/05/05/526750174/why-taste-buds-dull-as-we-age.

husband and I were first married, we were working around the house and he asked me if I was hungry for lunch. I looked at my watch and replied "yes." Puzzled, he asked why I'd looked at my watch and I realized at that moment that if it was between 11:30 a.m. and 1:00 p.m. I'd "allow" myself to be hungry for lunch, since that was generally lunch time. This was the first clue to me that I'd lost touch with hunger signals, as well as satiety.

If you're like me, you might be slightly horrified by the amount of food you feel you need in the beginning. This is because you can eat a whole lot of vegetables and starches before you feel full. Don't be alarmed if you're eating twice as much as you used to. Two full plates of salad and a bowl of soup may seem like more than you're used to eating, but calorically it's a lot less dense than a bowl of creamy Alfredo pasta or a slice of pizza. In my first 17 days of eating this way I couldn't believe how much I was eating. I also couldn't believe, when I got my bloodwork back, that my cholesterol had dropped 50 points in the same amount of time.

You may have emotional ties to certain foods, or foods you eat at certain holidays that you feel you can't give up. Your mom's cake that you always have for your birthday or your grandma's pie recipe for Thanksgiving might be things you decide to indulge in. Or, they might be things you decide to tweak and make healthier. Was Friday night pizza a tradition? There's no reason it shouldn't continue. We now put homemade pesto on pizza crust along with chopped green peppers, mushrooms, roasted garlic, onions, and tomatoes and top it with cashew cheese (and sometimes No Evil Italian sausage, sliced and browned). We enjoy pizza that tastes amazing and leaves us feeling amazing, rather than bloated and gassy and thirsty from all the salty cheese.

Speaking of cheese, a word here about it. Initially I thought giving up meat was going to be hard. Turns out for me, the smell of meat barbequing is mouthwatering, but the actual meat part, not so much. I've never been a huge steak fan. I liked turkey and bison burgers for a while, and I used to love pepperoni, olive, and mushroom pizza, but giving those things up really didn't feel like much of a sacrifice.

Cheese, on the other hand, was incredibly hard. Once I read about cheese and why it is so addicting, it made much more sense. Dr. Neal Barnard describes this in his book *The Cheese Trap*. He refers to cheese as "dairy crack," because in many ways it operates in the body just like a narcotic, triggering the brain to cry out for a fix.[115]

I felt a sense of relief learning that cheese is literally addicting. The dairy proteins act as mild opiates, and attach to the same brain receptors as heroin and other narcotics. Despite the fact that cheese has been tied to heart disease, "Americans eat 35 pounds of cheese a year…cheddar and its cheesy counterparts are the No. 1 source of saturated fat in the SAD," says Dr. Barnard.[116] So, while giving up cheese is hard (for good reason), it's definitely doable.

Marketing for you to be SAD

Admittedly it is hard to make changes in doing anything, but it's especially hard to eat differently than those around you. From commercials touting pizza with over a pound of cheese on them to

---

115 Neal Barnard, *The Cheese Trap: How Breaking a Surprising Addiction Will Help You Lose Weight, Gain Energy, and Get Healthy* (New York: Grand Central Life & Style, 2017).

116 "The Cheese Trap," *The Exam Room Podcast,* podcast, January 24, 2018, MP3 Audio, 59:42, https://www.pcrm.org/news/exam-room-podcast/cheese-trap.

milk posters adorning the walls of the elementary school cafeteria, it seems we're confronted with the SAD everywhere we go. This is not by accident. The macaroni and cheese boxes at the grocery store that are placed at eye level with Disney characters on them so your child sees them? That's not by accident either.

It's one thing to have advertisers constantly pitching junk food, but quite another to have doctors who've had, if they're lucky, one class on nutrition in all their medical school training giving you what they think is good nutritional advice. (Dr. Atkins, a cardiologist for goodness sake, promoted a high protein and high fat diet.) Ask your doctor about their training in nutrition and how many nutrition specific classes they took in medical school.

Do your homework when it comes to finding out the truth about nutrition "facts." In *The Future of Nutrition*, Dr. T. Colin Campbell points out that 55 percent of Americans take prescription drugs and many people take dietary supplements as well.[117] "In 2017, the average American's out-of-pocket pharmaceutical costs (including those covered by insurance) amounted to a shocking $1,162."[118] Pause to think about why we pay the highest prices on the planet for prescriptions. As Bernie Sanders once pointed out, the pharmaceutical industry has over 1,500 lobbyists on Capitol Hill for the 535 members of Congress.[119] You can be sure they're not lobbying for the availability and affordability of fresh fruits and vegetables for the American public.

---

117 T. Colin Campbell and Nelson Disla, *The Future of Nutrition: An Insider's Look at the Science, Why We Keep Getting It Wrong, and How to Start Getting It Right*, (Dallas: BenBella Books, 2020), 17.

118 Matej Mikulic, "Global Pharmaceutical Industry-Statistics and Facts," Statista, September 10, 2017, https://www.statista.com/topics/1764/global-pharmaceutical -industry/.

119 @berniesanders, Twitter post, October 21, 2021, 5:52, https://twitter.com/ berniesanders/status/1451305292067586089.

And remember, doctors, supplement companies, pharmaceutical companies, and nutrition fad promoters make a lot of their money off people making poor health decisions. The 2020 avocado advertisement during the Super Bowl aside,[120] there historically hasn't been a lot of money spent on selling whole plant-based/ HAPPY foods.

It's also hard to not do what everyone else is doing. It's easier to go along with the crowd. We're social creatures, and at times doing what everyone else is doing serves us well. At other times it's meant high-heeled flip flops seemed like a good idea. But while the trend for women to wear high-heeled flip flops was soaring, there were also those who chose to wear Crocs. Full disclosure, I personally made fun of Crocs until I tried them on and promptly bought a pair. For me, the comfort far outweighed looking unfashionable. Looking fashionable just wasn't worth sacrificing the comfort of Crocs. Thankfully, eating differently is having a moment these days. It is being met with less disdain and social outcasting than it was in the past. Plus, like Crocs, it feels way better.

My kids found the middle school years through freshman year in high school to be the hardest. Even friends would make fun of what they were eating, or daily say, "Ew, what's that?" But then things changed. In high school, friends would look at what they were eating and say, "Ohh, that looks so good. Can I try it?"

Sadly, you'll likely run into similar situations with adults. People can feel threatened when others are making new choices. You can choose to engage politely, offering your personal reasons

---

120 Qreativ, "Funny Super Bowl 2020|Avocados from Mexico Ad ft. Molly Ringwald," YouTube video, February 6, 2020, 1:10, https://www.youtube.com/watch?v= ZPCtVBCBunc.

for eating differently or a statistic, or you can simply smile and take another bite knowing your HAPPY meal (or food choices) won't be a source of scorn for long.

Help, I got off track, how do I get started again?

About a decade ago, Nathan George, the founder of Trade as One, "an online fair-trade company that uses consumer spending to create jobs for some of the most disadvantaged people in the world,"[121] was living in Santa Cruz and offered a challenge called Hungry for Change. We heard him speak and were inspired to give it a go.

Hungry for Change challenged you to eat what many people around the world subsist on daily for five days and then to donate what you would have spent on food and drink to the program of your choice (in 2012 this was estimated to be $15 a day). In the box we purchased, we received a bag of oatmeal, a bag of rice, and a bag of black beans. We could have black coffee or black tea (which more people consume worldwide), and we could add things like onion, green peppers, and spices to flavor our beans if we chose (though many people don't have the luxury of choosing). Otherwise, for five days we were to eat like the rest of the world.

As I recall it worked out to about a cup of oatmeal for breakfast and a cup and a half of beans and rice for lunch and dinner. It was shockingly sparse, and plain, and made us increasingly grateful for the amount and variety of food we enjoy each day.

---

121 Nathan George, "Making Money, Spending Money: What Do We Owe the Poor?" Stanford University, accessed February 26, 2022, https://web.stanford.edu/group/ivgrad/povertyforum/nathan-george.html.

Our daughter, who was 10 at the time, took her rice and beans to school for lunch (along with some fruit) and when classmates asked, told them what we were doing and why. Soon after, she started playing an educational game online where when she answered correctly rice would be given to children in impoverished nations. What a win-win!

We all gained appreciation for the daily variety of fresh fruits and vegetables we so casually enjoy after doing Hungry for Change. And in the future, when we found ourselves tired of our go-to meals, or missing old favorites, or were simply tired of meal planning, we'd do our own version of Hungry for Change and eat rice and beans for a few days until we were grateful and motivated again to make good choices.

You don't have to be this drastic if you don't want to be. Take a step back and evaluate why you "fell off the wagon." Were you tired, out of time, out of good food options, in a hurry? Decide what you'd like to do differently. Possibly that looks like having more healthy options prepped and ready to grab, or eating a snack mid-morning so you're not ravenous by lunch when tempting fast food is nearby. Whatever you do, don't beat yourself up. Take a deep breath, and begin again right away.

Now that you know what you're up against both internally (those pesky taste buds will change) and externally (billions of dollars spent advertising SAD foods), next we'll look at some proven strategies for staying on track and living HAPPY.

For fork's sake, LET'S DO THIS!

- Really taste your food the next time you eat. Take a deep breath before you start your meal. Try closing your eyes while you take your first bite. Notice what flavors and tastes jump out at you. Have any of your preferences changed?

- Make a plan for what you'll do if and when you get off track. Remembering that shaming yourself won't help, what will you do? Eat rice and beans for a day? Potatoes and broccoli? How will you work with yourself and remind yourself of the benefits of a HAPPY lifestyle?

- Watch the hilarious Douglas Lisle give a TEDx Talk on the Pleasure Trap, and how it can be avoided (17 minutes): https://www.youtube.com/watch?v=jX2btaDOBK8[122]

---

122 Tedx Talks, "The Pleasure Trap: Douglas Lisle at TedxFremont," YouTube video, 17:09, December 4, 2012, https://www.youtube.com/watch?v=jX2btaDOBK8.

DAY 6

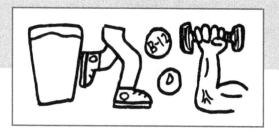

ADDING MORE COULD MEAN LESS

"Simply cutting down on the meat you eat to less than an ounce or two a day can dramatically reduce greenhouse gas emissions. In terms of land use, a more healthful diet, like a Mediterranean diet, may decrease your footprint by about a quarter, whereas even more plant-based diets can drop it by 50 percent or more."
—Dr. Greger[123]

WHAT'S THE HARDEST habit to break? The most recent one you're trying to overcome. Which is why I bring this up. Way back on Day 2, I asked you to accomplish the great clean out. If you followed my suggestion to the letter, I have to give you credit. That wasn't easy.

---

123   Michael Greger, "Which Diets Have the Lowest Carbon Footprint?" video, 5:56, November 18, 2020, https://nutritionfacts.org/video/which-diets-have-the-lowest-carbon-footprint/.

Unfortunately, I have a sneaking suspicion that maybe, just maybe, you didn't completely do it. You got rid of some particularly egregious SAD food—like blue cheese dressing that expired a month ago or that plastic baggie with some mini chocolate bars from Halloween 2006. You may have held onto some items just until you could find a replacement.

If you were overwhelmed thinking about facing empty kitchen cupboards, don't despair, there's another road to the same destination: adding in one HAPPY food at a time to replace a SAD item. Clearly, I think you will see results and feel better sooner if you commit fully, but it can be a tough transition and slowly substituting one food for another can work.

If you pick one SAD food item or meal a day to replace with a HAPPY substitution, you'll have replaced seven SAD items in a week. For instance, this week, swap out fast food with packing a HAPPY lunch. Instead of packaged cookies or desserts, give a homemade HAPPY dessert a try. Instead of replacing the boxed cereal you finish with more boxed cereal, give oatmeal a go. Or batch cook some soup and eat it for seven meals. You choose what works for you, just make sure you make a choice and take the next step of putting it into action.

This book is about making the jump to HAPPY in 10 days. If you can't fully make the jump by 10 days, you should have a plan as to when you're going to complete the move and hold yourself accountable. If you're getting stuck when it comes to actually making a change, review why you're doing this. Is it your health? The health of your family? The health of the planet? If making a change forever feels too overwhelming, then tell yourself you're just going to give this HAPPY thing a try for 10 days. Or, just for today you're going to try it. And then tomorrow, tell yourself the same thing.

Sometimes, the little kid in us starts trying to run the show. Take a moment to pause and figure out what is holding you back. Is there a younger version of you that is scared or feeling threatened by making a change?

Maria, a woman I worked with, described being a part of the "clean plate club." Growing up she had to finish her plate before being able to leave the table, so the thought of having to finish a plate of food she might not enjoy was daunting. Once she realized what was going on, she was able to tell herself she'd try the HAPPY meal she'd made, but if she didn't like it, she had the freedom to be finished whenever she wanted. Just giving herself permission to think differently about how she ate made a big difference.

Charles was having a hard time giving up eating out. As a child, eating out was a special treat and now that he was an adult and had worked hard and was able to eat out whenever he wanted, he didn't want to give up that luxury. Just becoming aware of the feeling of possibly missing out helped him realize it wasn't actually the food he was missing, but the idea of treating himself when he'd worked hard. He chose to continue to eat out occasionally, but found ways to "treat" himself other than with restaurant food.

Jean loved to create elaborate meals for her family and friends. She was nervous that cooking this "simply" wouldn't be as tasty or impressive to her foodie friends. She started with some elaborate appetizers the next time she had friends over—endive leaves filled with hummus, garnished with olives and fresh herbs, a HAPPY charcuterie board with dried fruits, fresh berries and apples, nuts, and homemade HAPPY cheeses. The amazed responses convinced her that she'd still be able to be creative and satisfy the tastes of even those who were still eating the SAD way.

If you're having a hard time getting going, just pick one thing to change today. Make one HAPPY choice, and when you've followed through with it, congratulate yourself for making a good decision.

My own additions and subtractions

For years, most mornings, I woke up before the kids in order to have some quiet time to myself: Time to read, pray, or meditate, enjoy a cup of coffee and a few deep breaths before the busyness of the day started. While my husband usually wakes up chipper and ready to tackle the day with a smile on his face, I somewhat stumble to the kitchen, bleary eyed, to make coffee before uttering cohesive words.

I'd read about the benefits of starting the day with some warm lemon water, and decided to try to start my day that way. It was an easy habit to start, since nothing was in my way in the morning and all I had to do was heat some water, and either squeeze half a lemon, or add some lemon juice to my glass of good intentions. This habit took just the amount of brain power and will power that I have first thing in the morning. It was easy to be successful with it.

The key is to pick something simple and doable that you can add to your daily routine. As discussed earlier, you can also start by subtracting one food a week that you know you'd like to eliminate, but for a lot of people that feels negative: it helps them to think of adding something instead.

Many people I've worked with in starting this lifestyle have given up salt, oil, sugar, caffeine, and alcohol, only to discover that strict limitations meant they felt they couldn't make this truly a lifestyle change and instead treated it more like a diet, eventually going back to most of their old ways of eating. Like many in the plant-based community, I haven't given up sugar or salt entirely. I still enjoy my cup of coffee in the morning and I occasionally drink wine or beer (though I have gone through periods of giving up both caffeine and alcohol). Remember, we're not trying a diet, we're making HAPPY and healthy lifestyle choices for the long-term.

So, pick something to add to what you eat this week. It could be something specific, like adding greens to one meal a day. Or to every meal: spinach in a morning smoothie or kale in a breakfast scramble, salad with lunch, and sautéed kale or chard added to dinner, for instance.

Or maybe a piece of fruit before lunch and dinner, or a glass of water before each meal. Pick one thing to add and try each day to make this a new part of your routine. Once you add a few things, you might find it easier to let go of some other things that aren't serving you anymore.

Vitamin B12

Another necessary thing to add, if you're cutting out animal products is vitamin B12, which is produced by bacteria found in the soil. Typically people get it from eating meat (because the animals eat plants directly from the soil with dirt on them). Our store-bought produce is clean these days, and even if you grow your own veggies or buy them with dirt clinging to them from the farmers market, you're still going to need to take vitamin B12

(Nutritionfacts.org suggests for adults under 65 at least 2,000 mcg cyanocobalamin a week, or 50 mcg daily). You cannot replace B12 by eating dirt, so please don't do that.[124]

Take a minute and think about something you'd like to add or subtract from your next meal. Pick something doable—something you already have on hand—and start there. Add that glass of water while you make dinner, or have that piece of fruit with breakfast. Feeling successful with one "add" will encourage you to do another. If you always have your phone on you, then set a reminder until it becomes habit.

Next, add to your grocery list something HAPPY you'd like to make a part of your eating habit. Fruit, greens, or whole grains are some good starters. Swaps like brown rice for white rice, or whole wheat flour for white flour are easy choices as well. Step up your game big time with adding a new HAPPY recipe.

Or, give something up, if that's your jam. Replace that bowl of ice cream after dinner with a walk or a plank or a piece of fruit. Stop eating fast food. Quit having butter laden popcorn with your movies. Give up added oil, especially vegetable oils (canola, corn, olive, palm, safflower, coconut…) since they aren't helping us.[125]

Pick a dietary habit that is doing more harm than good and experiment to see what life is like without it for a while. You'll likely find your newly improved digestion, clearer skin, and lack of body odor will be reasons enough to stick with being HAPPY.

---

124 "Vitamin B12," Nutritionfacts.org, accessed February 26, 2022, https://nutritionfacts.org/topics/vitamin-b12/.

125 T. Colin Campbell, "Plant Oils Are Not a Healthy Alternative to Saturated Fat," T. Colin Campbell Center for Nutrition Studies, updated January 7, 2019. https://nutritionstudies.org/plant-oils-are-not-a-healthy-alternative-to-saturated-fat/.

What about vitamin D?

Depending on your bloodwork, where you live, the color of your skin, and how much time you spend outside, you might be told you need to start taking vitamin D. Our bodies create vitamin D from direct sunlight on our skin. People with darker skin pigmentation require more exposure to ultraviolet radiation than do people with lighter skin. This is because while the melanin pigment absorbs ultraviolet radiation (UVR) and protects the underlying skin from damage caused by UVR, it also reduces the UVR available for vitamin D synthesis in the skin.[126]

On average, most people can get the vitamin D they need with 10 to 20 minutes in the sun daily. Pioneer doctors in WFPBNO (Dr. McDougall, Dr. Esselstyn and Dr. Greger) have thoughts on this and it's worth a quick Google search to see what they have to say.

These are all topics you should discuss with your doctor after seeing your blood work results.

Reward yourself (with something other than food)

George Throop was walking across America in honor of his late mom and inspiring other people to get out and walk in 2009. He stayed with friends of ours as he came through town, and we walked a few miles with him after having breakfast together. Our kids, after walking three miles asked if we, too, could walk across America. After some deliberation, we made a chart and told them that if they walked 30 miles we'd take them to "The Jungle," their favorite indoor play space which was about 30 miles away. We

---

126 Michael Holick, "Sunlight, Ultraviolet Radiation, Vitamin D and Skin Cancer: How Much Sunlight Do We Need?" *Advances in Experimental Medicine and Biology* 624, (2014): 1-16, https://pubmed.ncbi.nlm.nih.gov/25207357/.

made a chart, and the kids started asking to walk everywhere: to the park, to town, to the library, to school. They each took turns coloring in a box representing a mile when it was complete.

We thought the kids would lose interest, but they completed those 30 miles in less than three weeks. And when they finished, instead of losing interest, they asked if they could "walk" to Disneyland. We calculated it was 364 miles away, and this time drew a huge chart (again with boxes so they could color in each mile), and added a "treat" every 30 miles, like a movie, or Top-A-Lot Ice Cream (this was before we were a WFPBNO/HAPPY family). Though it took months, they did it, and we kept up our end of the deal and drove to Disneyland—reminding them as we drove that they'd actually "walked" that far!

If it helps, do something similar and make yourself a 10-day chart. Think of an incentive that will work for you. For some, a smiley face drawn on the calendar is enough to remind them that becoming HAPPY is helping them achieve maximum health and helping the planet to boot. For others, a check each day for completing the desired addition might mean giving themselves the gift of a leisurely soak in the tub, or watching a movie, buying a new item of clothing, or putting money aside toward a Vitamix. Short term rewards for long term goals can be great reminders to stay on track. Just make sure those rewards aren't foods you're trying to avoid, or in the end you've defeated the purpose!

Maybe you'd like to add watching or reading something inspiring to remind yourself why you're on this journey for the health of your family and the planet. I've worked with several people who committed to watching documentaries weekly or reading success stories of others who have made the switch from SAD to HAPPY to help keep the reasons for making the switch fresh in their minds. (I've listed several in the final chapter to get you started, if documentaries are of interest to you.)

You can keep adding to your knowledge of the HAPPY lifestyle. Take a few minutes to explore whatever questions you have. Research some answers. Adding to your understanding and knowledge can help thwart less-than-ideal choices when it comes to changing what you're eating.

Help, I'm eating WFPBNO/HAPPY but I'm gaining weight!

It's common to get tripped up here. People give up bacon and eggs for breakfast and replace it with toast with peanut butter. Or they swap out their cheeseburger and fries for a deep-fried veggie burger with sweet potato fries. Instead of steak and potatoes they order a vegan macaroni and cheese bake at a restaurant. At a quick glance these look like HAPPY swaps, but they aren't all whole foods or minimally processed either. So, while they might be vegan, they're calorically dense replacements.

If you don't need to gain weight, but suddenly find that you are, this little thing called calorie density might be at play. We'd been eating WFPBNO for years, but even though we'd cut out animal products and I was exercising, I couldn't get rid of the extra 10 pounds I was carrying. I realized the nut butter and avocado I was thickly spreading on my toast were partially to blame. As Dr. McDougall famously says, "The fat you eat is the fat you wear."[127]

---

127   Dr. McDougall Health & Medical Center, "The Fat You Eat, Is The Fat You Wear," YouTube video, 57:01, February 25, 2016, https://www.youtube.com/watch?v=-KBicWwnCdg.

Sure, it wasn't animal fat, but I was eating a lot of fat in the form of cashew cheese, nuts, and seeds. As soon as I changed to eating fewer calorie-dense foods (cutting out the nuts, nut butters, avocados, seeds, plant-based crackers, breads), the weight started to come off effortlessly. These foods aren't bad, but I now eat them in moderation.

Understanding calorie density is key to eating to satiety and not gaining weight. Instead of a handful of nuts, which is around 200 calories (we're talking 22 peanuts, 22 cashews, 29 almonds, 10 pecans, or 8 walnuts),[128] you could instead enjoy two bananas, three peaches, two apples, 50 strawberries, 24 orange slices, two and a half cups of pineapple, 60 grapes, or almost two and a half cups of blueberries. A cup of brown rice is also about 200 calories, a[129] medium baked potato (6.1 ounces or 173 grams), including the skin, is 161 calories.[130]

The fiber and liquid in food helps fill up your stomach and make you feel full. Starches, in addition to fruits and vegetables, are your friend here. If you're feeling hungry, reaching for some fresh fruit or even a baked potato or a cup of rice will likely make you feel more full than 10 pecans will, even though calorically they are similar.

Batch-cooked soups are really helpful, as is having a pan of baked potatoes or sweet potatoes, or some cooked brown rice on hand. When you get hungry, pull some out, add your choice of seasoning: mustard or ketchup, soy sauce or chili sauce, and you've just given yourself a nutrient-dense rather than calorie-dense snack.

---

128 "This Is What 200 Calories of Nuts Look Like," Daily Burn, updated July 2017, https://dailyburn.com/life/health/nuts-calories-serving-size-infographic/.

129 "Brown Rice," My Food Data, accessed February 27, 2022, https://tools.myfooddata.com/nutrition-facts/169704/wt1/1.

130 Atli Arnarson, "Potatoes 101: Nutrition Facts and Health Effects," March 7, 2019, www.healthline.com/nutrition/foods/potatoes.

COMPARING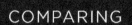

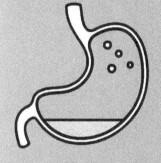

400 CALORIES OF OIL

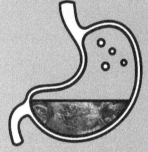

400 CALORIES OF MEAT

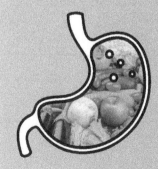

400 CALORIES OF VEGETABLES

Small tweaks can make a big difference. Instead of a banana or apple with peanut butter, just have the fruit and hold the nut butters. Instead of avocado on toast, have a baked potato or sweet potato topped with mustard or ketchup (Sounds gross? Don't knock it until you've tried it! It's become one of our favorite snacks!) Used to crackers dipped in hummus? Replace the crackers with veggies. Instead of ice cream, chocolate, or candy, try cutting up fruit, or putting a dollop of plant-based yogurt on top of cut fruit.

Remember, your taste buds are changing. Give them a little time to adapt, and you'll be surprised at how amazing real food tastes. (If weight loss is your goal, you might want to check out Jeff Novick's YouTube talk titled, "Calorie Density: How to Eat More, Weigh Less and Live Longer."[131]) There are no "bad" HAPPY foods, but you may just need to adjust the amounts of certain calorically dense foods if you find yourself gaining weight.

Keeping what you now know about calorie density in mind will help you avoid gaining weight from over-eating calorically dense foods and will help keep you on track by instead eating a variety and abundance of nutritionally dense, satisfying foods. Remember, you shouldn't be hungry eating HAPPY. If you are, then have some more HAPPY food!

Your family may have watched you making healthy choices and jumped on board, no questions asked. Or maybe they are watching and worried that next you're going to get rid of the TV and laughter. How exactly do you get your family on board? Next, we'll look at how to get family buy-in when it comes to making changes in the way we eat.

131 Jeff Novick, "Calorie Density: How To Eat More, Weigh Less and Live
     Longer," YouTube video, September 13, 2016, https://www.youtube.com/
     watch?v=0CdwWliv7Hg.

For fork's sake, LET'S DO THIS!

- Make a list of what you'd like to add to your meals. Start today, adding something or subtracting something if that's your jam.

DAY 7

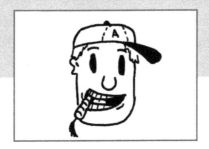

PLEASING KIDS, AND HOW TO SURVIVE YOUR SHOCKED PARENTS

So, you've added or subtracted something from your usual dietary routine, good for you! You're already making some healthy changes and choices. Maybe you're the only one in your family willing to make the change from SAD to HAPPY. That's okay. In time, after seeing all the positive changes in your health, others may be curious and want to join you.

Or maybe you're the primary caregiver and shopper and cook in the family and you'd like everyone to jump on board. If you'd like this HAPPY lifestyle to work for the whole family, you're likely going to need some buy-in. If you're worried about serving a HAPPY meal to your picky family, you're not alone. There are ways around and through this—let's look at some tactics that have worked for others.

I don't think my kids will eat that

"Why do we have to have white broccoli again?" my son commonly asked when he was young, upon seeing cauliflower on the dinner table. Though our kids ate what we did for dinner, it wasn't always without issue. For some reason, soup with chunks of vegetables was always a battle with my son. Even though he liked some of those same vegetables when not in soup, a bowl with a mixture of vegetables in liquid ignited a battle and tears.

One night I asked him to close his eyes, then I'd give him a bite of soup and ask if he could tell me the vegetable he was eating. For some reason he loved this, though he only guessed the vegetable correctly about half the time. What, only moments before, had been a struggle to get him to eat five bites (his age at the time), turned into his wanting to play "the soup game" for the rest of the meal. Thus began the game that almost always accompanied soup with vegetable chunks, for what seemed like a decade, but was probably less than a year.

If you've been making separate meals for yourself and your kids, I'm going to invite you to make life easier and stop doing that. Your kids are going to get all the necessary macro and micro nutrients they need from eating a WFPBNO/HAPPY diet. They will follow your lead and try new things if you are open to trying new things. I'm assuming you're sitting down as a family to eat dinner together. If not, now is the time to start. There's a lot of research showing how beneficial eating dinner together is.

This may be a new way of doing things, and all new things take a little time to get used to. But there are some tricks to employ here: kids love games, so how about making dinner about some games?

You could try to eat the rainbow for dinner, challenging yourself to cover every color of the rainbow as food options. How about some raspberries, radishes, or beets for red. Carrots, sweet potato, orange pepper, yellow pepper, or golden potato for orange and yellow. Green lettuce, snap peas, green pepper, and blueberries for the rest of the rainbow. "I spy with my little eye something red to eat. Does anyone else have anything red to eat on their plate?" As simple as it sounds, young kids eat this up (literally).

Has your child seen a rabbit or guinea pig eat? You could encourage them to "nibble like a rabbit" on their veggies, or chew and chew and chew like a cow chews its cud. Show them a video of bunnies or guinea pigs eating veggies, and pretend to be animals when you eat your veggies together.

Or, as we sometimes resorted to, you could take the number of bites of your age (so a five-year-old would take five bites, and a 35-year-old, 35 bites). Or try the "close your eyes guessing game," like we played with soup.

Distraction of a different sort can help too—how about a jar with questions. Each dinner, someone gets to pull out a question and you take turns answering it. This doesn't have to be fancy—write out questions and put them in a mason jar, or in an empty cup. I used this list that a teacher created, and added some of my own:

https://momastery.com/blog/2015/04/24/key-jar/[132]

132   "The Key Jar: 48 Questions to Ask Your Kids," We Can Do Hard Things with Glennon Doyle, April 24, 2015, https://momastery.com/blog/2015/04/24/key-jar/.

Questions, such as, "What was your first thought when you woke up today?" or "If you could switch places with one friend for a day, who would it be?" or "What's the best thing about living here?" get minds racing. When you're hungry, and also thinking and listening and conversing, you tend to eat what is in front of you.

Or go with our standard: high, low, and what the heck. Each person tells of a high, a low and a what the heck moment from their day. For instance, one child might say their high was playing in the park after school. Their low was falling off the swing at the park. And their what the heck was when they swallowed their tooth that fell out at lunch at school (true story from one of our kids). Usually, while talking and listening to each other, our kids would eat with only an occasional reminder that they needed to take a bite.

Invariably there will be things your kids don't want to try. We had a "no thank you helping" in our home. So, even if someone didn't want to try something, a "no thank you helping" meant they got a little bit to try, and that was all. Research completed by Healthy Families British Columbia found it takes 12 times of trying a food to develop a taste for it.[133]

So, maybe the first time you serve a beet it doesn't sound good to your two-year old. That's okay, and very normal. You could ask them to smell it, and describe what it smells like. Or move it around and see how it makes the plate red. Next time you serve it, you could dice it, or roast it, or grate it, and have them touch it and see how their fingers turn red. You don't have to have beets every night for 12 nights. But know that it will take some time for acquired tastes to become acquired. This also goes for adults. You

---

133   Cat Bowen, "Surprise: Your Kid Needs to Try a Food 20 Times Before You Can Give Up," Romper June 17, 2019, www.romper.com/p/how-many-times-does-a-child-have-to-try-a-food-before-they-like-it-more-than-you-think-17999317.

didn't love asparagus as a child? Have you tried it recently, cooked several different ways?

It goes without saying that you will eat when you are actually hungry. So, if the kids have been snacking on goldfish crackers or string cheese an hour before dinner, they probably won't be that hungry to try HAPPY minestrone soup. However, if they had some whole fruit as an afternoon snack and were running around playing until dinner time, there's a greater chance they'll be willing to try some new foods.

Obviously, I'm not saying don't feed your kids when they're hungry. I'm saying be cognizant of what and when they are eating. You could try the broccoli test as well. Next time you feel hungry, ask yourself if you'd eat a cup of raw broccoli. If the answer is no, then you're probably not hungry. You may actually be bored, thirsty, lonely, or tired instead.

Having a bowl of ready-to-eat fruit (apples, bananas, oranges) out at all times is great for kids. You could have an area or a drawer in the fridge that is deemed the snack section. Enlist the kids to help decide what could go in there, then have them help cut up veggies and fruit so they're ready to grab whenever the kids are hungry. This helps them have buy-in and cuts down on the time they stand at the fridge with the door open looking for something to eat.

Making sure your kids (and you) are being active will also help on this journey to health. Hopefully, they are behaving like kids and are running around and jumping and playing and danc-ing. If not, put on some music while you're cooking dinner and make it a dance party to get excited for dinner together. Or take a walk as a family either during the day or after dinner.

How strict do we need to be?

At first, we were black and white and tried to eat WFPBNO/ HAPPY 100% of the time. We quickly found it nearly impossible to eat out or eat at a potluck or at friends' houses for dinner without throwing in the towel, or worse, throwing caution to the wind and eating our hearts out.

For instance, around this time our son attended a party and consumed six hot dogs and 12 cookies—he was in fourth grade! We quickly realized that the all or nothing approach wasn't working very well. So, we transitioned to a "we eat this way at home" plan, so that when we were out or with others we could enjoy whatever we wanted, and not feel pressure that we had to eat any certain way.

Initially this eased the self-imposed pressure, but it eventually led to eating out or parties or potlucks becoming an excuse to eat what we'd been missing (namely cheesy, fatty foods). I bit my tongue as my husband and kids ordered pepperoni pizza, and cringed as they got real ice cream cones, but soon a funny thing happened.

After indulging in all those "treats" we'd been missing out on, we'd experience stomach cramping and gas and feeling bad in general. This was because, after not eating animal products, our bodies had stopped producing the enzymes needed to break them down. I purchased enzymes to take before eating at a restaurant or others' homes where we couldn't eat WFPBNO/HAPPY. (It wasn't until years later, while doing research for my certificate in plant-based nutrition, that I learned that these were mostly acting as a placebo.)

As the months went on, eating out became less and less of an excuse to splurge, and we all started ordering vegan options at restaurants—not because we were guilted into doing it, but because in the end we felt better eating that way. The true miracle occurred a few years later, when my son was going to a birthday pizza party. Before dropping him off, I asked him if he'd like to take an enzyme so his stomach wouldn't hurt. "No, I'd rather not, because this way I'll only have one piece because my stomach will start to hurt, but if I take the enzyme I'll eat way more." My elementary school aged son had come up with his own self-regulating plan.

Help! The parents or grandparents are coming over!

I'd noticed the last time I saw my dad that he had a few memory lapses that seemed new. Living two states away, we go months between visits and any changes seem pronounced. After learning about the effect of diet on brains (mainly due to amyloid plaque buildup) I asked my mostly pescatarian mom, who was the cook in the house, if she'd be willing to try cooking WFPBNO/HAPPY. She agreed and I booked a flight to Washington to surprise my dad for his 76th birthday.

As my gift, I bought *The Starch Solution* by Dr. John McDougall[134] for my dad, and printed out recipes from the free 10-day McDougall program online, along with some of our WFPBNO /HAPPY favorites and put them in a ready-to-use binder. I cleaned out their refrigerator, removing the Vegenaise, Ranch, and Thousand Island dressings, and both the shredded and block cheeses. I removed the tortilla chips and crackers from

---

134 John McDougall, *The Starch Solution* (Emmaus: Rodale Books, 2013).

the cupboards. I went shopping, stocked up on items needed for the recipes, and made oil-free hummus, chopped veggies, and a few meals to put in the freezer. I encouraged my parents to give this a real try for at least 10 days and notice whether they felt any different. I cooked meals while I was there, and encouraged them as best I could.

Months later, on a visit, my mom returned some of the things I'd bought for them saying that they'd sort of tried them, but they knew we'd use them. As much as I wanted better health for both of them, I couldn't do it for them.

How *do* you introduce family and others to WFPBNO when visiting? Do you have some new favorite, go-to meals in your family now—HAPPY nachos, pasta, enchiladas, lasagna, chili—that your kids love? These would be great to introduce to others when they come to visit. When the grandparents see their grandkids enjoying healthy food that will help them grow without contributing to health risks, they are sure to be proud.

Once, when my in-laws were visiting from Washington, we prepared dinner. After we'd been eating for a few minutes, my father-in-law asked what type of green beans we were eating, as they were good but pretty chewy. We all had a good chuckle after explaining they were edamame (soy beans), and you just eat the inner bean, not the outer skin he was chewing on. Unbeknownst to us we'd introduced him to edamame, but not very well!

Parents and grandparents may need an explanation as to how you are getting all the nutrients you need—after all, their generation grew up with different norms around eating (Fruit cake,

Spam, Carnation Instant Breakfast, and Jello salad, anyone?). Emphasize your reasons for doing this—this is where your blood-work results can be especially helpful, as there's a good chance that older family members will want to lower their cholesterol or blood pressure or insulin levels as well.

Remember, not too long ago you thought all of this was a load of hogwash too, so be kind. If nothing else, most people will eat a meal that is prepared for them, so they'll get to try something they might not have had otherwise. Or, you could prepare the meal and not mention at all that it's a HAPPY meal. When they comment on something they liked, or ask about some part of the meal, then you have your chance to tell them what you're trying.

If you're like me, you want to share all the information you've learned about the SAD, and pass on all the amazing benefits to eating HAPPY. You might want to share what you've learned about the planet and the way our food choices impact the health of the planet. Depending on your family, maybe they'll be recep-tive. More often though, new ways of being are met with hesitancy and distrust or downright disbelief.

People feel threatened when someone starts doing something differently. If that's the case, you can simply say something like, "We're trying this new way of eating, and we'll see how it goes." Family members may feel less threatened by that, and over time, by watching you thrive, may eventually warm up to the idea and ask some questions.

In explaining to the grandparents/friends/co-workers what you're doing, you might be able to speak to the fact that you don't have to wear deodorant anymore, or that your gas doesn't smell, that your skin has never been clearer, and that it even seems like your nails are growing faster. Okay, so you might not want to share all these details. But nonetheless, they might be things you're already experiencing on day seven.

For fork's sake, LET'S DO THIS!

- Print out the questions from https://momastery.com/blog/2015/04/24/key-jar/[135] and stick them in a jar to use at dinner tonight. Let someone pick one question for discussion at dinner. Tomorrow night, someone else gets to pick the question.

- Ask the kids what HAPPY foods they'd like to have on hand for snacks. Have them help wash or slice the foods and put them in an easy-to-find place for HAPPY snacking.

- Pick one of your family's newest favorite HAPPY meals to make and share the next time family comes to visit.

DAY 8

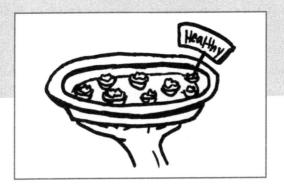

WHAT ABOUT EATING OUT?

EATING AT HOME is almost always going to be the healthiest and easiest choice. But sometimes it just isn't an option. Whether you are required to eat out with others, or simply want to enjoy a meal at a restaurant, what follows are ideas for making it work and keeping it HAPPY.

A cautionary note about eating out: it's nearly impossible to eat out without eating oil. You can ask that your dish not have oil added, but in my experience most restaurants can't/won't accommodate cooking with no oil. So, just know that when you eat out you will most likely be eating added oil.

How to eat out at restaurants/business meetings/potlucks takes a little getting used to, but is easier than you may think.

HappyCow is an app for finding vegan food nearby. Or if you're ordering out you can use Grubhub or DoorDash to search for vegan options. You can order pre-made plant-based meals to be delivered to your home from businesses like MamaSezz (mamasezz.com), or pre-packaged meals from Leafside (goleafside. com)—both have been helpful for us at different times.

Even if you don't utilize those types of options, you can easily make a meal from a standard restaurant menu. Most restaurants have vegetarian options, so you can always order something off that menu and ask them to hold the cheese.

Almost every restaurant has salads that can be modified. Order a salad and ask if you can add fresh or steamed or cooked vegetables on top or as a side. Same goes for a baked potato, or pasta. Order a few veggie sides à la carte to make a meal.

Don't be shy about asking for different elements of other meals. For instance, I recently swapped egg-noodles for house-made potato gnocchi at a local Italian restaurant. Or I'll take cheese and meat off something and ask to substitute avocado or tofu, or just all the veggies they have.

When in doubt, you can tell them that you have a medical condition and need to keep animal products and extra oils out of your food. They will usually work with you. It can help to call ahead and ask about options, so they're prepared when you arrive. (Be sure to leave a nice tip to thank them for their willingness to work with you.)

In an Italian restaurant you can order pasta with meatless red sauce and vegetables. Or make your own calzone or pizza without cheese. Some restaurants have raviolis filled with mushrooms or spinach or other veggies instead of cheese. Angel hair pasta with pomodoro sauce, or any pasta with sauteed veggies and garlic work well. (Pastas in traditional Italian restaurants may contain egg. Ask if they have a whole-wheat pasta, or an egg-free option.)

Italian restaurants are usually up to their ceilings with piles of bread. Find the brownest version of bread and dip it into red sauce.

In a Mexican restaurant, you can order a veggie burrito or avocado enchiladas or veggie fajitas. Even sides of rice and beans and corn tortillas with some salsa and guacamole work great—make your own burritos to taste. A few people I know bring their own homemade oil-free chips to Mexican restaurants so they can have chips and salsa before their meal with everyone else. Another woman just asks for some plain corn tortillas and dips those in salsa instead of oil-laden chips.

Most Chinese, Thai, Korean, sushi, and Indian restaurants have a variety of vegetarian dishes that are whole food, plant-based friendly. I usually don't mess with the no oil part when eating out, unless they are drizzling oil on something, then I ask for it to be left off.

Here are some of my specific recommendations:

- Chinese restaurants: Fresh (not fried) veggie spring rolls are a great start. Look for veggie dumplings and wontons. Noodle dishes often are made without meat by substituting tofu or veggies.
- Thai restaurants: Fresh spring rolls and soups can be found without meat or dairy. There are many noodle dishes and curries that are HAPPY, as well as salads.
- Korean restaurants: Stir-fried noodles, fermented vegetables, tofu stew, and rice dishes all can be made HAPPY.

- Sushi restaurants: You can keep it simple with a cucumber or avocado roll, or many sushi restaurants have elaborate veggie sushi options to choose from. Edamame makes a great side, and sometimes you can find a HAPPY miso soup.

- Indian restaurants: The spices in Indian food are incredible, as is the amount of oil used. That being said, there are a lot of HAPPY dishes to choose from—from chana masala to dal tadka, tofu paneer, and mulligatawny soup to some types of naan.

- Poke Bowl restaurants: Making your own poke bowl makes it really easy! Start with brown rice or zucchini "noodles" as your base, and pile on the veggies. Pick from oil-free sauces (shoyu, soy sauce, ponzu) to keep it HAPPY.

- Vegan restaurants: These can vary from junk-food vegan to high-end whole food plant-based. Look for dishes that are as whole as possible (so a homemade black bean, mushroom, and grain burger would be a healthier choice than an Impossible or Beyond Burger, which are highly processed. A grain bowl or salad or sandwich piled with veggies would be healthier than nachos with vegan cheese and vegan sour cream).

- Vegetarian restaurants: Depending on the restaurant, you may have lots of options. Look for dishes that you can omit dairy from to make them HAPPY. As with strictly vegan restaurants, try to avoid highly processed vegan versions of food and go with whole, plant-based options instead.

I have to go to a work conference, HELP!

If you're attending a conference for work, it can be worthwhile to call ahead and ask about vegan options for meals. If it is to be buffet style, you can usually find oatmeal and fruit, or potatoes or toast to make a WFPBNO breakfast. Depending on the choices, a salad with lots of toppings or a sandwich for lunch can usually be arranged.

Dinners can be tricky if you don't ask ahead. We've attended functions where the main choices were steak or fish, leaving us to eat the veggie sides and dry rolls as our dinner, which was less than ideal. So, do your stomach a favor and ask ahead of time what the options are.

One woman I know brings her Instapot and toaster everywhere she travels. She makes her toast in the morning, makes soups and cooks grains in the Instapot and never worries about not being able to be HAPPY. While this can work when traveling for pleasure, if you're attending a working meal, do yourself a favor and inquire about the options beforehand. If there's absolutely nothing you can eat, ask for hot water and add it to a HAPPY meal replacement (McDougall cups of soup work well here, as well as LeafSide meals), which can easily be packed in a suitcase.

Eating at a friend's house and how to navigate potlucks

We never expected friends to cook something different for us if we were invited over to eat. We decided when we started our HAPPY journey to be good guests and to eat whatever anyone served us. But when friends learned what we were doing, they started calling ahead and asking what we could eat. We assured them we'd eat what they cooked and that we were happy even to bring our own food if that made things easier, and that we did not expect them to cook differently for us. But being nice people, many of them opted to take the opportunity to try a new HAPPY

recipe. I hope you have such nice friends, and that your joining
them at their home for dinner gives them a chance to try out
something HAPPY.

If not, you can decide to eat whatever is being served, or offer
to bring a side or another dish to share that you know you'll be
able to eat and that they just might try and enjoy as well. Pasta or
quinoa salads work well. A potato bake casserole dish, or HAPPY
baked macaroni and cashew cheese are also crowd pleasers. Making
a dish people are familiar with that looks like something they'd
usually eat is helpful here. HAPPY lasagna is hard to tell apart
from SAD lasagna, as is baked HAPPY mac and cheese. People are
usually more apt to try something they at least recognize.

Professional WFPBNO chef and author Christopher Carnrick
says he brings *The Starch Solution* (one of Dr. McDougall's books
on eating WFPBNO) as his hostess gift whenever he's invited over
for dinner. He also brings a plant-based dish to share, with recipe
cards already printed so people can grab one and take it home with
them.[136]

Attending potlucks can also be an opportunity to bring some
new food choices to the table. What I bring usually depends on
time and the group. If I have extra time, maybe I'll make something a little more involved, especially if I think the people attending the potluck might be open to trying new things. You can
go all out and make pan-roasted portobello steaks with lobster
mushrooms and charred veggies for a HAPPY take on surf 'n turf,
or prepare a butternut squash bisque or individual HAPPY pot
pies. You can opt to bring homemade carrot dogs to throw on the

---

136 Carnrick, Christopher. "Cooking with Christopher Carnrick." (12-Day McDougall
     Program, August 2021).

bbq, try making HAPPY ratatouille, homemade HAPPY sushi or make an herbed nut cheese to share.

If, on the other hand, I'm pressed for time or I'm quite sure no one will give WFPBNO deviled eggs or kale cake a try, then I won't waste my time making it and I'll bring a hummus, cracker, and veggie plate or colorful quinoa salad instead. You can always bring something you enjoy—that way you know there will be at least one option you can eat. I would advise making more than you think is needed. Often by the time we get food at a potluck, the HAPPY dish we brought to share is all gone!

Here's a HAPPY recipe below that is great for sharing.

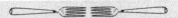

HAPPY deviled eggs

Buy six to eight egg-size potatoes (both red or yellow work). Wash, then boil the potatoes until cooked (depends on the size of your potatoes, but a fork should go in them easily, approximately 10 minutes). Drain, and let cool. When cooled, cut the potatoes in half and use a spoon or a melon baller and scoop a hole out of the middle (it now looks like a boiled egg without the yoke). Place the scooped holes in a bowl and mash. Add 1/2 cup hummus, 1-2 Tbsp relish, or chopped dill pickles, 1 Tbsp of mustard, 1/2 tsp each of garlic and onion powder, and mix (you can add sriracha if you like it spicy...we usually do half and half). Fill the holes with the potato/hummus mixture, then sprinkle some smoked paprika on top. Try not to eat them all before sharing!

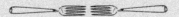

What the heck do you eat for dessert?

It can help to make a dessert or treat of some sort to show people that you aren't giving up enjoying food, and that you're not surviving on just beans and rice. There are many WFPBNO/HAPPY desserts to choose from. A simple Google search will give you recipes for things such as sweet potato brownies, chocolate mousse made with tofu, wicked chocolate pie, lemon bars, and carrot cake, in addition to the black bean brownies, kale cake, and HAPPY peanut butter ball recipes you can find on my website. You may choose to make a special dessert, serve it and then—after your guests are surprised how good it tastes—you can tell them what's in it.

A really simple Snickers bar-like dessert starts with a date sliced down the middle, with the pit taken out. Fill the pit area with a small spoonful of almond butter. Place a chocolate chip on top of the almond butter. Stick it in the freezer to chill (or freeze to pull out for later consumption).

For fork's sake, LET'S DO THIS!

- Make and share a new WFPBNO meal or dessert. Bonus points for sharing it with someone.

DAY 9

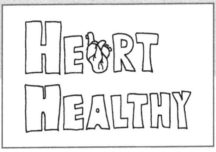

WHAT DO I TELL OTHER PEOPLE? (WHAT TO RESPOND WHEN PEOPLE ASK WHY YOU'RE DOING THIS)

WE WERE FEELING so good after making the switch from SAD to HAPPY that we wanted to tell everyone how they, too, could make some simple changes and feel incredible. We quickly realized that talking about diet is like talking about money, sex, or religion. It turns out many people are very uncomfortable talking about what they eat and why.

We didn't want to come off as preachers, we wanted others to experience the benefits of good health. Bumbling our way through a myriad of conversations, we learned a few helpful ways of talking about this sensitive topic.

One useful tactic to try is memorizing a statistic or quote to have at the ready. When someone invariably asks why you aren't having a hamburger or steak at the neighborhood bbq, you have a prepared answer to give. For example: "Even the academy of nutrition and dietetics says that a well-rounded vegan diet is healthy and that vegetarians and vegans of any age and at any stage of life do better insofar as preventing obesity, type 2 diabetes, cancer, stroke and heart disease.[137] Or you could just show them your T-shirt that says, "Strokes Suck!". Or mention my new favorite quote by the past-president of the American College of Cardiology, Dr. Kim Williams: "There are only two kinds of cardiologists: those who are vegan and those who have yet to read the data."[138] I've mentioned this one before, but it's too good not to say again!

In my experience, sometimes people are genuinely interested in hearing what you have to say. At other times, people immediately become defensive and want to explain to you why they eat the way they do. These days, this usually includes some well-intentioned but highly unscientific story of someone they've read about or know who lost 25 pounds in a month eating keto.

You'll be amazed by how many people you know are suddenly medical experts, dishing out advice on the amount of protein you should be consuming or supplements you should be taking. Many will insist that the latest fad diet (keto, paleo, Mediterranean) is helping them or someone they know. You can

---

137 Vesanto Melina, Winston Craig, and Susan Levin, "Position of the Academy of Nutrition and Dietetics: Vegetarian Diets," *Journal of the Academy of Nutrition and Dietetics* 116, no.12 (2016): 1970-1980, https://pubmed.ncbi.nlm.nih.gov/27886704/.

138 Rich Roll, interview with Dr. Kim Williams, podcast audio, November 5, 2017, https://www.richroll.com/podcast/kim-williams/.

feign shock and with a surprised voice say, "And all this time I had no idea you were a medical doctor with a specialty in nutrition!" Or, simply smile and nod if you're not looking for confrontation.

After these kinds of exchanges, I can feel inadequate in wanting people to know more truth, but I've learned that not everyone wants to learn more or do better. Or maybe just not right now, and that's okay. It's their journey not yours.

An alternative route you might take is to tell interested listeners your own personal health reasons. When you explain that your doctor is concerned about your cholesterol levels and this way of eating is working to lower those numbers, there's nothing to argue with. When you tell someone you're no longer having to take insulin, or are off your blood pressure medication, people's ears perk up.

These days, bringing concerns about climate change into the conversation makes a lot more sense to people than it used to. CO_2, methane, and the deadly runoff from subsidized CAFO's (Concentrated Animal Feeding Operations) are no longer fringe topics. The rainforest being razed for cattle or for growing palm oil are topics that are more mainstream.

You could also just tell people about the amazing dinner you enjoyed last night, or how you're so surprised that your child is asking for snap peas for a snack, or about how much money you've saved on groceries this month.

At the end of the day, it's you and your family and the planet's health that is of the utmost concern. So, if Bob in accounting makes fun of your new way of eating while snacking on his Slim

Jim beef stick, so be it. If neighbor Jane says she just can't survive without her steak and lobster and cheese, let her arteries be the ones to eventually teach her the truth.

Your friends may have some questions they'd like to ask. These are common ones:

Why didn't my doctor tell me this?

Your doctor or pediatrician is a smart and caring person, I'm sure, but they may have had only one nutrition class in all their medical training. This may be new information to them. Remember, as recently as the 1950s, doctors were recommending cigarettes to their patients.[139] This was not because they wanted them to get lung cancer and die. Rather, at that time, based on the information they had, they thought they were making wise recommendations.

Maybe your doctor has experienced a lot of patients unwilling to make dietary changes and patients asking for pills as solutions to their health problems. You could very well be the first person to suggest WFPBNO as a viable treatment option to your doctor. They may not have heard of Dr. T. Colin Campbell, Dr. Caldwell Esselstyn Jr., Dr. Neal Barnard, Dr. John McDougall, Dr. Dean Ornish, or Dr. Michael Greger, to name a few.

If your doctor isn't receptive to you changing to a scientifically proven way of bettering your health, you can look for a new doctor. Or, you can do what many people have done and show them what a WFPBNO diet can do by being a real-life example.

---

139 Leah Lawrence, "Cigarettes Were Once 'Physician' Tested, Approved," Healio, March 10, 2009, https://www.healio.com/news/hematology-oncology/20120325/cigarettes-were-once-physician-tested-approved.

What about keto/paleo/low-carb/South Beach/ Mediterranean diets?

Your coworker across the hall went on a keto diet and started doing CrossFit and lost 50 pounds. Your mother-in-law is eating no sugar and doing Weight Watchers and has lost seven pounds. Your good friends eat paleo now and say they feel better than ever. A fitness coach you know swears by intermittent fasting. Everywhere you turn, news/magazines/social media are talking about the latest trend in eating.

The thing about diets and trends is that most of them usually work—for a time. However, we're not looking for a quick fix or the next trend to inform our eating. We're basing our eating habits on long-term health and sustainability, both for us and the planet. We're adopting a new way of eating that will help us (and the planet)—in both the short term *and* the long term.

As someone who dieted off and on for years, I get the lure of trying a new diet. What we're transitioning to though isn't a diet but rather a lifestyle choice that we'll be able to maintain for life. In other words, we're running a marathon, not a sprint. It's not the occasional departure from eating HAPPY that is going to make or break us. Instead, it's the many daily decisions and habits that will count in the long run.

Besides, six months from now, I'm guessing your keto coworker or family member on Weight Watchers will be back to where they were, or worse. Not because they lack discipline or didn't try hard enough. But rather because what they were doing wasn't sustainable long term. You can feel good about giving up trying to follow the latest food fad. You can rest assured that eating

HAPPY means you won't ever have to research the next big diet fad to see if you should try it.

There will be another diet trend to come along. "The staggering truth is that the diet industry is a $60 billion per year industry with a 95 percent failure rate," says Amber Karnes, founder of Body Positive Yoga and creator of Body Positive Clubhouse.[140] As people rush out to buy new products to replace things they've stopped eating, you can keep eating all the whole, plant based, minimally processed HAPPY foods you want.

But I thought carbs make you fat

Carbohydrates in general have gotten a bad rap. Sure, if you're eating vegan simple carbohydrates like white bread, doughnuts, French fries, and potato chips, you're likely to gain weight and your health will suffer. But what we're talking about are complex carbohydrates (this is where the "whole" part comes into the "whole foods plant-based no oil" way of eating).

As the Mayo Clinic describes,[141] metabolism is the name we give to the body's process of converting what we eat and drink into energy. Your body needs energy for things it does even at rest, such as breathing, repairing cells, and circulation. If you have more muscle, you burn more calories. If you're a male, you typically burn more calories than a female of the same age and weight, due to having more muscle. And as you age, you typically lose muscle therefore slowing down calorie burning.[142]

---

140   Amber Karnes, "Shocking Facts About the Diet Industry," Body Positive Yoga, accessed February 25, 2022, https://bodypositiveyoga.com/shocking-facts-diet-industry./

141   "Metabolism and Weight Loss: How You Burn Calories," Mayo Clinic, November 10, 2020, https://www.mayoclinic.org/healthy-lifestyle/weight-loss/in-depth/metabolism/art-20046508.

142   Ibid.

Eating and food processing (technically called thermogenesis) use about 10 percent of the carbohydrates and protein you take in. All that digesting, absorbing, storing, and transporting of food takes energy.[143] Physical activity accounts for the rest of the calories your body burns up each day, making it the most variable of the factors that can determine how many calories you use. Unless you have a medical problem that slows metabolism, such as having an underactive thyroid gland or Cushing's syndrome, you probably can't blame your metabolism for weight gain.[144] The basic equation of eating more calories than you burn is what commonly leads to weight gain.

While some people seem to lose weight easier than others, we all lose weight when we burn more calories than we eat. Those who seem to lose weight more easily may just be more physically active throughout the day—not only by working out, but even by doing things such as gardening or housework or possibly even fidgeting.

So what do carbs have to do with all this? Carbohydrates, fats, protein, and water are the basic nutrients our foods contain, and are referred to as macronutrients (as opposed to vitamins and minerals, which are called micronutrients). These nutrients are what our bodies need for growth, repair, and maintenance. "Carbohydrates are the body's most efficient way to get everything it needs," says Dr. John McDougall.[145]

Carbohydrates are produced by plants in photosynthesis and are commonly called sugars. When the sugars attach together to make a long branching chain of molecules they're called complex carbohydrates, or commonly, starch. When we eat starch,

---

143 Ibid.
144 Ibid.
145 "A Lesson in Nutrition," Dr. McDougall Health and Medical Center, updated April 11, 2013, https://www.drmcdougall.com/articles/nutrition/lesson-in-nutrition/.

or complex carbohydrates, enzymes break down the chains into simple sugars that pass easily through our intestinal wall into the bloodstream to be distributed to all the cells in our body. Metabolic processes then convert these simple sugars into energy. The dietary fiber present in all plants assists in regulating the body's use of sugars and helps to keep hunger and blood sugar in check.

Fats give structure to cell membranes and store energy. They don't dissolve in water because of their chemical structure and are not as easily digested as sugars. Because proteins provide the raw materials for a large part of the functional and structural components of our bodies, they are only used as a source of energy as a last resort.[146] You've heard of marathoners "carbo loading" the night before a race? This is so that they have the energy their body can quickly retrieve when needed.

While we don't want refined white sugar to be a major part of our diet, whole fruits with all their natural sugars and fiber are fine. Same goes for refined wheat flour—instead, enjoy whole wheat, so you're getting the bran and fiber, which helps to slow the absorption of the sugars. In short, when eating WFPBNO/HAPPY you don't have to worry about counting calories, adding up micro or macro nutrient amounts, or weighing your food. You eat when you're hungry to satiation. It's that simple.

As Dr. McDougall points out, carbohydrates (starches) have been what most civilizations have lived on for the past 14,000 years. Rice in Asia, corn in Central America, potatoes in South America, and barley and wheat in Europe were the basis of most of the calories consumed in these populations.[147] Not that they didn't eat other types of food,

---

146 Ibid.
147 "Fat or Carbs: Which is Worse?" Dr. McDougall Health & Medical Center, updated October 23, 2013, https://www.drmcdougall.com/articles/nutrition/fat-or-carbs-which-is-worse/.

but carbohydrates provided the bulk of their calories. The same is true in healthy populations today. The Japanese are among those with the longest average life expectancies, and among those who eat the greatest amount of carbohydrates. This diet ensures they have the lowest incidence of heart disease and diabetes.[148, 149]

Staying as close as possible to whole foods (and away from processed foods) is what we're aiming for. Say you used to eat a plain bagel with cream cheese. Now you can enjoy a whole grain, oil-free bagel with hummus, cucumber, red pepper, red onions, roasted garlic, and arugula. Or a bowl of brown rice with all the same ingredients on top. Eating similar types of foods is possible, even when switching to WFPBNO/HAPPY.

Beyond your immediate and even extended family, this good thing needs to be shared! How will you help share the news?

For fork's sake, LET'S DO THIS!

- Find a quote to share about why you're making this switch.
- Order a "STROKES SUCK!" t-shirt and let it do the talking for you.
- Learn what happens in an open heart surgery.
- Find out what happens during a stroke.

148 Kirti Pandey, "8 Things the Japanese Do that Helps Them Live Longest: Study Looks into Food, Attitude, Habits that Influence Longevity," November 18, 2021, https://www.timesnownews.com/health/article/8-things-the-japanese-do-that-helps-them-live-longest-study-looks-into-food-attitude-habits-that-influence-longevity/832947.

149 Kirk Spitzer, "Secrets from the Longest-Living Place on Earth," AARP, May 2014, https://www.aarp.org/health/healthy-living/info-2014/longevity-secrets-from-japan.html.

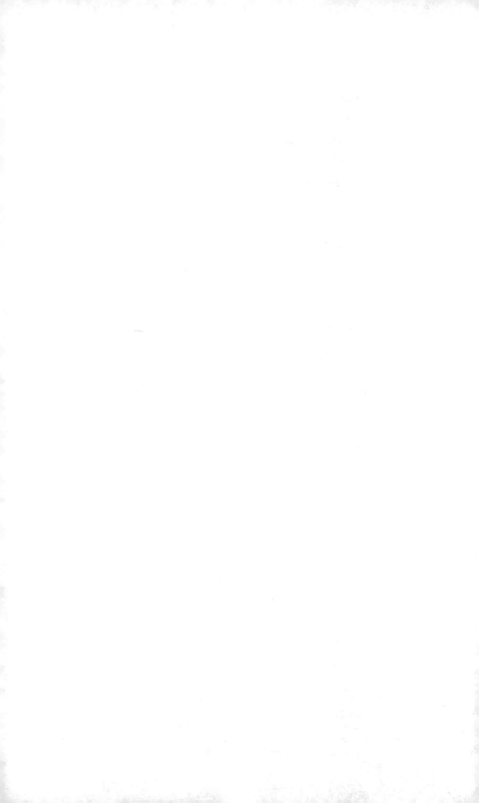

DAY 10

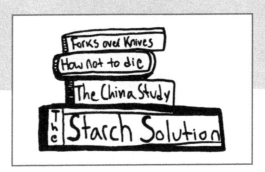

HOW DO I KEEP THIS UP?

"Each year more people by far die of chronic diseases caused by a bad food system than have died of coronavirus, but we don't treat it as a national emergency. Why? Because chemical companies, food companies, and big agricultural companies make trillions of dollars off that system."
—Marianne Williamson[150]

OVER A DECADE ago we went camping in Yosemite for the first time with friends. We were all blown away by the huge walls of rock, and enjoyed hiking and seeing waterfalls and wildlife and biking around the valley floor. One night we decided to go to Curry Village where there was a pizza place with outdoor picnic tables. While waiting for our pizza we sat down at a table and one of the

150 @marwilliamson, Twitter post, March 28, 2021, https://twitter.com/marwilliamson/status/1376238114952318984.

biggest, fattest squirrels we'd ever seen promptly ran out of the surrounding woods and onto the deck where the tables were. On the table was a sign that said, "Please don't feed the squirrels. They are wild and fare better eating natural foods. Eating pizza and other human food has caused weight gain, hair loss, and other illnesses including death." Looking around us at the people waiting for pizza or finishing their cheeseburgers, we all had to agree it wasn't just squirrels who were being affected by the human food, but the humans as well.

Now twelve years in, our family has lowered cholesterol and literally reversed heart disease (as evidenced by removed plaque visible on our carotid artery tests). We recently received a perfect score on a calcium test (an X-ray test of the heart that helps detect and measure calcium-containing plaque in the arteries). This is despite coming from families with heart disease, cancer, and diabetes.

Encouragement in the form of success stories have been very helpful for me. To know there are other individuals and families out there who have made the transition successfully and are thriving is helpful and encouraging on days when cooking or staying on track doesn't sound all that fun.

Examples of other success stories and encouragement help me when I feel overwhelmed or under supported in choosing to live a HAPPY lifestyle. While I'd love to tell you my family of origin has fully adopted this way of eating, they haven't. But several friends over the past 10 years have. One of them even teaches plant-based cooking classes at a community college now. Many of our kids' friends have also changed how they eat as well. Countless other couples and families around the world have made the switch from SAD to HAPPY and are thriving.

I've guided many people through the decision to try living HAPPY for a bit—just to lower their cholesterol, or get off blood-pressure medication, or lose some extra weight they'd been carrying around. But a month in, they felt better than they had in years. Their lipid blood panel numbers improved, they got off medications, their excess weight came off without any effort, and they decided to stick with this new way of being, even though they'd never intended to.

Dear reader, I hope that if the motivation from your original "why" fails you at times, you'll find other enjoyable side effects from choosing to be HAPPY that will spur you on. Some tried and true motivation in the way of books, documentaries and websites can also help steer you back on course if you've momentarily lost your way. Here are some of the many ways to keep up the motivation:

MOVIES/DOCUMENTARIES:

I recommend starting at the top and watching one a week. Head to my website for eight more suggestions.

Forks Over Knives[151]

This is the film that started it all for many people in 2011. If you're going to watch one film on whole food plant-based eating, this is probably the best eye-opening overview. Roger Ebert of the *Chicago Sun-Times* gave the film three out of four stars and wrote: "here is a film that could save your life."[152]

---

151 *Forks Over Knives,* directed by Lee Fulkerson (United States: Virgil Vilms and Entertainment, 2011), DVD.
152 Roger Ebert, *"Eat meat and die!"* May 11, 2011, https://www.rogerebert.com/reviews/forks-over-knives-2011.

The Gamechangers[153]

Debuting in 2019, this is another film that is a great one to start with. Elite athletes, soldiers, and scientists share about meat, protein, and strength. Plant-based doctors, as well as Arnold Schwarzenegger, James Wilks, Scott Jurek, and Olympic athletes and NFL players all talk about their experiences with making the change.

PlantPure Nation[154]

This film, released in 2015 by Nelson Campbell, son of T. Colin Campbell, follows three people as they demonstrate the health benefits of a purely plant-based diet.

Eating You Alive[155]

This film takes a practical look at why Americans are so unhealthy and how what we eat can improve our health. Featuring Samuel L. Jackson and leading nutritionists and medical professionals such as Neal D. Barnard, Joel Fuhrman, Michael Greger, and Dean Ornish.

Cowspiracy[156]

A 2014 documentary exploring the impact of animal agriculture on the environment and investigating some environmental organizations such as Greenpeace, Sierra Club, Surfrider Foundation among others.

---

153 *The Game Changers,* directed by Louie Psihoyos, (United States, 2018), DVD, 1:26.
154 *PlantPure Nation,* directed by Nelson Campbell, (United States: 2015), digital, 1:35.
155 *Eating You Alive,* directed by Paul David Kennamer Jr. (United States: Gravitas Movies, 2018), 1:48.
156 *Cowspiracy: The Sustainability Secret,* directed by Kip Andersen and Keegan Kuhn, (United States: A.U.M Film, 2014), 1:31.

Orangutan video

(https://m.youtube.com/watch?v=TQQXstNh45g)

A 90-second cartoon produced by Greenpeace International high-lighting the effect of deforestation on orangutans. "Dedicated to the 25 orangutans we lose every day."[157]

BOOKS:

More suggestions can be found at www.forforkssakebook.com

The China Study[158] and *The Future of Nutrition*[159] by T. Colin Campbell, PhD

The Starch Solution by Dr. John McDougall[160]

The Healthiest Diet on the Planet by Dr. John McDougall and Mary McDougall[161]

Prevent and Reverse Heart Disease by Caldwell B. Esselstyn Jr.[162]

How Not to Die[163] and *How to Survive a Pandemic*[164] by Michael

---

157 Greenpeace International, "Rang-tan: The Story of Dirty Palm Oil," YouTube video, 1:30, August 13, 2018, https://www.youtube.com/watch?reload=9&app=desktop&v=TQQXstNh45g.
158 T. Colin Campbell, *The China Study: The Most Comprehensive Study of Nutrition Ever Conducted and the Startling Implications for Diet, Weight Loss, and Long-term Health* (Dallas: BenBella Books, 2006).
159 T. Colin Campbell and Nelson Disla, *The Future of Nutrition: An Insider's Look at the Science, Why We Keep Getting It Wrong, and How to Start Getting It Right* (Dallas: BenBella Books, 2020).
160 John McDougall, *The Starch Solution: Eat the Foods You Love, Regain Your Health, and Lose the Weight for Good!* (Emmaus: Rodale Books, 2013).
161 John McDougall and Mary McDougall, *The Healthiest Diet on the Planet* (New York: Harper One, 2016).
162 Caldwell B. Esselstyn Jr., *Prevent and Reverse Heart Disease: The Revolutionary, Scientifically Proven, Nutrition-Based Cure* (New York: Avery, 2008).
163 Michael Greger, *How Not to Die: Discover the Foods Scientifically Proven to Prevent and Reverse Disease* (New York: Flatiron Books, 2015).
164 Michael Greger, *How to Survive a Pandemic* (New York: Macmillan, 2018).

Greger, M.D., FACLM

WEBSITES:

Forksoverknives.com[165]

Forksoverknives.com has thousands of WFPBNO/HAPPY recipes and success stories. They cover health topics, have a cooking course, a beginner's guide and a meal planner.

Drmcdougall.com[166]

Drmcdougall.com has everything you need—thousands of recipes, information in the form of articles and videos on health issues, inspiring success stories, a Starch Solution certification program, and a free online program. They also have a 12-day online program I highly recommend.

Nutritionfacts.org[167]

Dr. Michael Greger has thoroughly researched information on anything and everything whole food plant-based and provides short videos and blogs on almost any topic or question you might have concerning eating plant-based. Wondering if fish is good for you? If you should get a mammogram? What about conflicting information on nuts or the keto diet or how much B12 you should be taking? He covers it all.

---

165 "Our Story," Forks Over Knives, accessed February 26, 2022, https://www.forksoverknives.com/our-story/.

166 "Our Story," Dr. McDougall Health & Medical Center, accessed February 26, 2022, https://www.drmcdougall.com/our-story/.

167 "About NutritionFacts.org," NutritionFacts.org, accessed February 26, 2022, https://nutritionfacts.org/about/.

Nutritionstudies.org[168]

This is T. Colin Campbell's Center for Nutrition Studies website and it has a wealth of information on what plant-based eating is, education/certification opportunities, articles published, recipes, a community to join, and a helpful newsletter you can sign up to receive (which has recipes, success stories, and the latest in plant-based eating).

SOCIAL MEDIA:

Instagram:

@forksoverknives[169]

@nutritionfacts.org[170]

@goplantstrong[171]

@themcdougallprogram[172]

@nutritionstudies

@dresselstyn[173]

@ripesselstyn[174]

@jane_esselstyn_rn[175]

@plantbasednews[176]

168   "About Us," T. Colin Campbell Center for Nutrition Studies, accessed February 26, 2022, https://nutritionstudies.org/about/.

169   Forks Over Knives (@forksoverknives), Instagram, accessed February 26, 2022, https://www.instagram.com/forksoverknives/.

170   NutritionFacts.org (@nutrition_facts_org), Instagram, accessed February 26, 2022, https://www.instagram.com/nutrition_facts_org.

171   PlantStrong (@goplantstrong), Instagram, accessed February 26, 2022, https://www.instagram.com/goplantstrong/.

172   Dr. McDougall (@themcdougallprogram), Instagram, accessed February 26, 2022, https://www.instagram.com/themcdougallprogram/.

173   Caldwell B. Esselstyn, Jr., MD (@dresselstyn), Instagram, accessed February 26, 2022, https://www.instagram.com/dresselstyn/.

174   Rip Esselstyn (@ripesselstyn), Instagram, accessed February 26, 2022, https://www.instagram.com/ripesselstyn/.

175   Jane Esselstyn (@jane_esselstyn_rn), Instagram, accessed February 26, 2022, https://www.instagram.com/jane_esselstyn_rn/.

176   Plant Based News (@plantbasednews), Instagram, accessed February 26, 2022, https://www.instagram.com/plantbasednews/.

@plantbasedjuniors[177]
@therealchefaj
@eatfortheearth2021

Facebook:

Forks Over Knives

Eat for the Earth Worldwide

Be an advocate

Be an advocate in your family. You have the opportunity three times a day—with breakfast, lunch, and dinner—to affect change for good in your family and for the planet. As we've been discussing throughout the book, keep using meals and snacks, shared dinners, and potlucks as ways to bring awareness and health to those you love.

How about at your kids' school? Advocate for healthy school food for your child and all children. Schools must meet certain requirements to receive reimbursement from the federal and (sometimes) state governments. Certain requirements are astounding—for instance that milk must be offered but does not need to be taken.

"It would literally take an act of Congress to change the fact that milk must be offered," says Amie Hamlin, MEd, Executive Director of the New York Coalition for Healthy School Food. "And what is really astounding is that there is no requirement for schools to offer non-dairy milk to accommodate lactose intolerant children or those whose families don't drink milk. This especially impacts BIPOC children, the majority of whom are lactose

---

177 Plant-Based Juniors (@plantbasedjuniors), Instagram, accessed February 26, 2022, https://www.instagram.com/plantbasedjuniors/.

intolerant." She goes on to say, "Research indicates that: those who consume the most milk as children may have the highest levels of colorectal cancer as adults; severe constipation in children can be reversed when they give up all dairy; dairy is associated with prostate and endometrial cancer, and that much of the population (the global majority) is lactose intolerant (a normal condition, as digesting milk after weaning is not natural)."[178] Check out healthyschoolfood.org for ways to get involved and help bring about change.

Advocate for yourself and your child with your doctor and pediatrician. Take a look at Physicians Committee for Responsible Medicine (pcrm.org) for resources on incorporating nutrition in medicine. Ask questions and share the information you're learning with your health care professionals. Best of all, show them with your increasing health and vitality how eating HAPPY is working for you.

Ask your favorite restaurants if they'd consider adding plant-based options, or doing a meatless Monday. A local burger restaurant we frequent has a meatless Monday option (a house-made veggie patty called Tracks in the Grass). On their board next to their menu options, they include an inspiring fact about going meatless one day a week, encouraging people to give it a try.

Beginning in the 2019–2020 school year, all New York City public schools (reaching 1.1 million students every week) went to Meatless Monday.[179] And the network of New York–Presbyterian

---

178 Amie Hamlin, "Advocating for Healthy School Food," T. Colin Campbell Center for Nutrition Studies, updated January 4, 2019, https://nutritionstudies.org/advocating-healthy-school-food/.

179 "NYC Expands Meatless Monday to All Public Schools," Monday Campaigns, March 11, 2019, https://www.mondaycampaigns.org/meatless-monday/news/nyc-expands-meatless-monday-schools.

hospitals (Allen, Columbia, Westchester, and Cornell sites) now provide vegetarian choices for their staff and visitors every Monday.[180] Mondaycampaigns.org even has a weekly feature called "Meatless Recipes to Help Your Children Eat More Vegetables" with recipes and ideas.[181] All these changes came about because a few concerned and committed people made requests and offered to be a part of the solution.

Contact food companies to tell them you love their whole food plant-based products that don't have oil and you'd buy more of them if they made more options. I've thanked No Evil and Upton's for products they've made, and asked Field Roast and various vegan coffee creamer producers to please make oil-free options. I've written Clif Bar to ask why they have to add palm oil and to let them know we'd love a no-oil bar made with whole, plant-based ingredients.

Be the squeaky HAPPY wheel. Companies want to sell products, and if their products aren't selling, they make changes. Request changes and vote with your dollar. Slowly, the attitude is changing toward the HAPPY way of eating. More people are choosing to eat more plant-based foods, which is driving companies to react to reach those consumers.

Involve others

For a little over a year, we joined with three other families and took turns cooking a meal a week (we divided it up so that

---

180 "Meatless Monday Arrives at New York-Presbyterian Hospital," Monday Campaigns, April 23, 2019, https://www.mondaycampaigns.org/meatless-monday/news/meatless-monday-arrives-newyork-presbyterian.

181 "Meatless Recipes to Help Your Children Eat More Vegetables," Monday Campaigns, January 25, 2021, https://www.mondaycampaigns.org/meatless-monday/meatless-recipes-to-help-your-children-eat-more-vegetables.

each family received two meals a week, or cooked once every two weeks to make it doable). It required a lot of effort the day we cooked—making enough food for four families, packaging it, and delivering it—but receiving delicious meals delivered to our door that we didn't have to cook made up for it.

See if a friend or a few friends would be up for trading WFPBNO/HAPPY meals. You'll get to try a variety of meals you might not have made for yourself and you'll probably be inspired to try cooking some new options to share, plus you'll gain friends to exchange recipes and information and new knowledge with. What a gift.

If you can't find anyone locally who shares your interest in eating HAPPY and helping the planet, then look online. PlantPure Communities has pods (plantpurecommunities.org). If there isn't one in your area, you can start one. Whole Communities (wholecommunities.nutritionstudies.org) is an online platform committed to building resilient communities of health through whole food, plant-based nutrition. Eat For the Earth (eatfortheearth.org) has a Worldwide Facebook group with meetings online once a month offering support for anyone interested in changing their diets toward more plants and fewer animal products.[182]

Start a Plants Only club and meet at a park after school where kids can play and parents can socialize and everyone can enjoy a HAPPY snack. Get creative or keep it simple, but research shows that we do better at completing goals when we choose specific actions to follow through on, and we do better when we do these things with others.

---

182 "Eat for the Earth," Facebook page, accessed February 25, 2022, https://www.facebook.com/eatfortheearth/groups/?ref=page_internal.

You've made some significant changes, and I'm sure you already have success stories of your own to share with others by now: how much your cholesterol has dropped, how much weight you've effortlessly shed, how much money you're saving on groceries, what your kids ask to eat...

How will you go about sharing what you've learned?

Staying the HAPPY course

Remember that the goal is not perfection, but greater health for yourself, your family, and the planet. Keep your personal "why" at the forefront of your mind. I was lucky enough to have a doctor who was open (and transitioning himself to a WFPBNO diet) but I was irritated that on the shelves in his office he had "healthier" choices for people to see—things like lower fat turkey slices. When I asked why he had these items, his answer depressed me, but over time made more sense. A lot of his patients weren't willing to go cold turkey (pun intended) and give up all the foods they'd eaten their entire lives, so he was presenting healthier options to switch to. I've come to understand that some people operate better this way—small, incremental steps can equate to lasting changes over time.

As a kid, I remember when my mom made the switch from the two-percent milk we'd been drinking for years, to non-fat. At first, non-fat milk tasted like colored water, and I didn't think there was any way I'd ever get used to it. But over time, it became normal. Maybe by switching from salami cold cuts to lower fat turkey slices some people become accustomed to change and then eventually make the swap to veggie sandwiches or tofu bon mi sandwiches.

My doctor no longer has the "healthier" food options on his shelves anymore. He does however, have books written by Dr. McDougall and Dean Ornish.

Staying HAPPY for life

We were driving down Highway 1 on our way to meet friends at the beach. My then-elementary age daughter was talking about what a friend had said about what type of man she wanted to marry. I listened, and then asked my daughter what she had said when her friend asked her what *she* wanted in a future husband. Her answer: "I don't want a man who brings home the bacon." I just about howled with laughter but was curious as to what she meant because I didn't know she was familiar with the saying. So, I asked her, "What do you mean? Why not?" "Because," she resolutely declared, "I want to be vegan when I grow up." Ahh, it all made sense now.

That little girl is now 20, and eating HAPPY. She's a sophomore in college and this year moved off campus to an apartment with three other vegans. My son, when looking at colleges as a senior in high school, made sure they had vegan dining options before making his choice. It hasn't been easy, but like most good things, it's been worth it. Both of my kids endured classmates making fun of what they had in their lunches, or commenting when they were sitting outside on the grass at school, "Why don't you just eat this, it's vegan," or mocking them when they decided to have a bite of something a friend had that wasn't vegan. But they also had friends who asked thoughtful questions and changed their eating habits. Friends who became vegetarian and vegan themselves over the years. And best of all, they are enjoying healthy bodies and are proud to be doing their part to help take care of our planet.

10 days to life: a SAD to HAPPY celebration of choice

You've made some huge changes that are impacting your health, your family's health, and literally the health of the planet. Way to go, you! If you haven't already, now is the time to learn to ask for what you need—at the grocery store, at your kids' school, at business meals. For the most part, I've found people to be very accommodating, especially when they know a little bit about why you're doing what you're doing (remember that quote you memorized to share with people as to why you're doing this, this is another place you can use it).

If your grocery store doesn't carry a fat-free hummus, or mayonnaise, or salad dressing, ask them to (you can suggest brands you've looked up that you'd purchase from them). Of course, you could just buy these from Amazon, but your local grocery store wants and needs your business, and you probably go there for other items as well. And just think, maybe there are others out there who, when they see an oil-free dressing/cracker/dip, will be willing to give it a try as well.

Take the seven minutes to call ahead to the business lunch or dinner to make sure there will be something you can eat and enjoy. You're paying for it (or your employer is), so it might as well be something you can happily eat. What once was an "out there" way of eating is becoming much more normal.

When we were visiting a friend in Copenhagen a couple years ago, she apologized that they didn't have as many vegan restaurants as we did in California, and then proceeded to take us to four amazing totally vegan restaurants in five days. And while we were there, we passed a McDonald's sign advertising a meatless burger. At McDonald's! (This was 2018, before the Impossible and Beyond Burgers were on any fast-food menus in the states.) Changes are happening all around us on the food front. If all else fails, use health reasons when citing your need for something different. "I'm combating heart disease and so can't have oil or animal products" is a true statement.

Dear reader, you've done it! You've learned what eating WFPBNO is all about, and why it makes sense both for your health and the planet's. You've learned through reading and through suggested actions what it takes to make the transition, and hopefully you're already reaping the rewards. You can do this. Your health and your family's health depend on it. The future of the planet depends on it. So have fun with it! Find new WFPBNO recipes online or in cookbooks. Invite friends and family to join you on the adventure. Stay HAPPY, friends!

For fork's sake, LET'S DO THIS!

- Check out some success stories on the Forks Over Knives website, or Star McDougaller's on DrMcDougall.com.
- Think about ways to keep yourself motivated.
- Did you do your blood draw? Remember those results.

ACKNOWLEDGEMENTS

Zach, thanks for the encouragement, the belief in me and for being my technical support always. Sophia and Jenison, thanks for eating whatever I cooked (mostly) without complaint, and for listening to me rant about factory farming, oils, and the industrial food complex. Dad, thanks for your support and for always cheering me on. Mom, thanks for playing devil's advocate on much of what I was learning, ensuring I did more research, and for always having a garden and fresh fruit and vegetables around.

Rod and Kathy Brown, though I'd never wish the circumstances on anyone, I'm impressed by the healthy changes you've made. Cheers to not feeding cancer cells.

To the people who volunteered to be early readers: Troy Jenison, Sophia Brown, Barb Neill, Julie Hills and Cory Caletti— thank you for your comments, your questions and your time. I value them all.

To friends who willingly ate HAPPY meals with us and listened to me share random facts, bless you. Peter Thomsen, those Mother Trucker burgers all those years ago were an experience in and of themselves. Jana Thomsen, John and Cory Caletti, Maria Cavigelli, Kurt Fitze, Kristina Trolle, Ken and Barb Neill, Rob and Lynn Wesson, Laura Bontrager, the Storrer family, among many others over the years.

David Smith, thanks for your support and encouragement in general. You always remind me of what is true. Liz Harley and Eric Lehman, your laughter and banter makes dark days brighter. Thank you Ruth Peterson, for the use of your awesome place in San Francisco when I needed an escape. Michael Ann Jacobson, the Monday morning runs have been a God-send, as has been your friendship and shared excitement.

Jens, thanks for doing the artwork, even when as a senior you had more exciting things to do, like surf or skate or mountain bike with friends.

Dr. Steven Leib, and sweet Vivian—thanks for all the years of helping to spread the good news about lifestyle medicine and for being open to change.

To my heroes in the WFPBNO world: Dr. T. Colin Campbell—your book, *The China Study* started it all for me. Your other books, and the plant-based nutrition certification are a testament to your dogged research which continues to educate and inspire. Dr. John McDougall, your dedication to telling the truth and helping others continues to be inspiring. Mary McDougall, your recipes made it not just possible but enjoyable for us, especially in the early days. Heather McDougall, Anthony Lim, MD, JD, Doug Lisle, PhD, Jeff Novick, MS, RDN, Christopher Carnrick, Jack Dixon, NSCA, CPT, Kori Burningham—you guys have nailed it with your work in the 12-day online program— thank you!

Dr. Caldwell Esselstyn Jr., your dedication to those who needed the most help and your willingness to walk with them continues to inspire confidence in whole, plant-based foods with no oil.

Ann Crile Esselstyn and Jane Esselstyn, thanks for sharing your recipes and wisdom and laughs with the world! Rip Esselstyn, your books helped cement what we were learning, and we were so relieved we could still have chocolate.

Dr. Michael Greger, your attention to detail is incredible. Thanks for all the research, and for sharing what you've learned with the world. Your grandma would be so proud.

Dr. Neal D. Barnard, Melanie Joy, PhD, Dr. Dean Ornish, Dr. Dean and Ayesha Serzai, thank you for your years of effort and work to help others.

Beth Love, thanks for founding the supportive Eat for the Earth (Worldwide and Santa Cruz) and for encouraging others on their journey.

Mollie Forest, thanks for the marketing help, even when on vacation in Maui!

COVID, you big jerk, I reluctantly thank you for time spent at home not working, without which I probably never would've tackled this project. And also for teaching the world what a co-morbidity is and reminding us all what our health is worth.

And lastly God, thanks for creating self-healing bodies and a self-healing planet, for fork's sake, please help us learn to care for both.

The Plant-Based Nutrition Certificate
from

 T. COLIN CAMPBELL
Center *for* Nutrition Studies

and powered by eCornell

is an online, video-based certificate,
featuring lectures from over 25+ leading
experts, including Dr. T. Colin Campbell.

Students will learn about the science
behind a plant-based diet, Dr. T. Colin
Campbell's 8 Principles of Food and Health,
the role nutrition plays in chronic disease,
including cancer, heart disease, diabetes,
Alzheimer's, and autoimmune disorders,
and much more!

To learn more visit:
nutritionstudies.org

and join the free Whole Communities here:
wholecommunities.nutritionstudies.org

EPILOGUE

Jenison Cut Out High-Fat Plant-based Foods and Lost 20 Pounds Effortlessly

The fundamentals of the McDougall Program are simple yet often difficult to implement. Star McDougallers have either adopted the Program themselves by learning from our website and books or joining one of our programs. For personalized help, learn more about the *12-Day McDougall Program*. For questions on whether a change in diet can help your ailment, learn more about our *consultations*.

Learn more

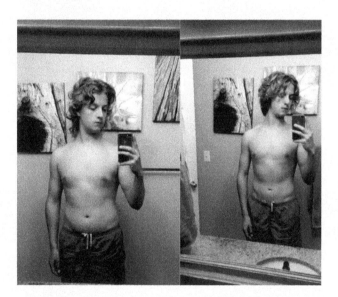

Our family has been eating WFPBNO at home since our son Jenison was 6 years old. This past August our family decided to do the *12-Day McDougall Program* as a refresher. Jenison and his older sister participated some, while we, his parents (and even grandparents a couple months later) enjoyed the course in its entirety. During the 12-day, we were reminded about calorie density. We opted to cut out extra fat (all the whole plant fats we loved and ate quite a bit of – nuts, nut butters, avocado and seeds). Since Covid had somewhat eased up (at the time) we'd also returned to some outdoor dining which was always vegan, but usually had oil. In addition, we had been enjoying homemade cashew cheese almost weekly, and had built up some 'insulation'.

Jenison, who was 17 at the time and just starting his senior year of high school, decided when he was out with friends to not eat high fat vegan foods – he'd usually have 'vegan' fast food, or food with oil and an occasional soda. Instead he decided to stick to veggie sushi or a bean burrito with just beans, rice and pico de gallo. Within 3 weeks he lost 15 pounds, and by around 5 weeks he'd lost 20 pounds. He was eating to satiety but enjoying much less calorically dense foods. His dad and I lost 15 and 12 pounds respectively, as well.

It was such a fun transformation to watch – Jenison really got it seeing the effects so quickly. He asked for articles to give to his friends when they would say they needed their protein shakes after a mountain bike ride or body surfing session together. He daily grabs a few pieces of fruit to have on hand to snack on at school. We've found eating out to be the slipperiest slope – there are more vegan options with vegan cheese or fake meats on pizzas or burgers, but less whole food plant-based options, plus all the oil. It's much easier to eliminate unwanted fat eating at home. We knew this before, we just didn't realize what a big impact it was having on us.

Now 18 and heading to college in the fall, Jenison has a much more personal understanding about what eating whole, plant-based foods with no oil can do for your body.

It hasn't always been an easy journey being the kid whose mom made smoothies and WFPBNO cookies for their friends, but for me to see them as adults choose to take good care of their bodies and the planet while spreading the word themselves is a true blessing.

Thanks for everything!

Rachael (Jenison's mom)

For more on how Jenison and his family made the transition, look for Rachael's book *For Fork's Sake: A Quick Guide to Healing Yourself and the Planet Through a Plant-Based Diet* coming out in September 2022 www.forforkssakebook.com.

9 798986 138015